H

Healthy Eating

Diana MacAdie

Based on the Tyne Tees Television Series

Stanley Paul, London

Stanley Paul & Co Ltd
3 Fitzroy Square, London W1

An imprint of the Hutchinson Publishing Group

London Melbourne Sydney Auckland
Wellington Johannesburg and agencies
throughout the world

First published 1977
© Trident Television 1977
© Drawings Stanley Paul 1977

Printed in Great Britain by litho at The Anchor Press Ltd
and bound by Wm Brendon & Son Ltd
both of Tiptree, Essex

I S B N 0 09 131260 4 (cased)
I S B N 0 09 131261 2 (paperback)

Drawings by Martin Williams

Contents

Acknowledgements

This book is based upon the Tyne Tees television series entitled 'Healthy Eating' and I should like to thank, in particular, its producer, Lisle Willis, who set this book in motion. I should also like to thank all those who contributed to the programmes, especially Professor Arnold Bender from the University of London, who has offered me invaluable advice during the writing of this book, Professor John Walker from the University of Newcastle and Anne Robertson, who is the dietician responsible for providing the dietetic services for the Newcastle Area Health Authority.

I am also grateful to Derek Miller from the University of London for his helpful comments, and, finally, to my publisher, Roddy Bloomfield, who has offered continual encouragement and advice.

The table on page 96 is based upon information supplied by courtesy of the Metropolitan Life Insurance Company, USA; most of the material in Appendix A is reproduced with the kind permission of the Controller of Her Majesty's Stationery Office; and, finally, the table in Appendix B is also reproduced with the kind permission of the Controller of Her Majesty's Stationery Office.

Foreword

Since everyone eats, and always has eaten, food, it is surprising that so little is known about it. Even among the sciences, those of nutrition and food science are among the newest, centuries after disciplines such as chemistry and physics.

Food, too, appears to be one of the most abused of our possessions – when it is available we eat too much of the wrong foods, or miss out on the right foods and, of course, sometimes maltreat it in the kitchen.

In the industrialized, western world, where food is freely available and costs us only a small part of our income, obesity is one of the major problems. Everyone knows how to lose weight – eat less – but few can do it and fewer can do it properly. Properly means getting enough of all those nutrients needed for good health, more than a dozen vitamins, more than a score of mineral salts, fats of various types, proteins and carbohydrates. When the slimmer cuts his diet by half he stands a good chance of cutting his intake of vitamins, minerals, and so on, by half and of suffering in consequence.

Even those who are not slimming may not be getting enough of all these nutrients. The trouble is that there is no rapid deterioration in health, no sudden result such as follows careless crossing of the road. Instead, there may be a very slow, insidious deterioration of one's health, infections may be more readily caught, bones may be more fragile, healing of wounds and recovery from disease may be slower. If this happened to you, you would not know that it was abnormal and certainly not know that it may have been due to sub-normal nutrition.

What, then, can one do? Improve your diet as an insurance policy, just in case it is deficient in something, a matter that would be difficult to prove. This can be done by making sure that all the nutrients required are present on the plate – proper selection of food and proper cooking.

Few people know what this means. That is why we need more information about what we should eat, what is in the packet, what the manufacturer is doing to our food, and what we are doing or should be doing with our food in the kitchen. What steps should the expectant mother take to ensure the best start in life for her baby? How should she feed her infant? Can you improve the health of the elderly by a better diet? Can some of the diseases of modern life — heart disease, obesity, bowel disease — be mitigated by diet?

There is no absolutely clear answer to these questions but there are precautions we can take, and these you will find in the contents of this book.

ARNOLD E. BENDER

Healthy Eating

1 The need to eat

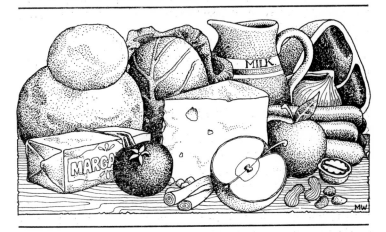

Eating is a joy for most, a duty for a few, but a necessity for all. The food we consume provides us with the raw materials that are needed for our growth and upkeep, and it also provides us with life-giving energy.

A century ago we knew little about what happens to our food once inside us, but now, with the tremendous advances that have recently been made in the science of nutrition, we know much more. For this reason we are, theoretically, in a better position to achieve a healthy diet – but this needn't be just one diet: many different diets using a wide variety of foods can all be given the title, 'A healthy diet'.

In this first chapter I want to explain the fundamental facts about diet, a knowledge of which is essential if you are to really understand the information in the other chapters.

I have split it into four parts. The first is a general outline of why you need to eat. The second is a description of the constituents and energy supplied by food in more detail. In the third I take a look at how much of everything is needed and what happens if you over or under-do the correct amount. Finally, I relate these needs back to the food you eat, and I explain how you can achieve a really healthy diet by following some very simple rules.

Why You Eat - In General Terms

The simple question, 'What are you?' may or may not be something you have ever asked yourself. If it is, then the answer must have surprised you.

The answer is anything but simple; that is, if it is given in complete detail. But I can make it a good deal easier for you by just supplying you with an outline.

The chemical make-up of the human body

Basically, you are a mass of different chemical elements — as, indeed, is everything you can touch — and the four main elements are oxygen, carbon, hydrogen and nitrogen. These are joined together in rather a special way to form such combinations as water or one of the many different proteins, which are then further grouped to give the highly complicated structure you know as the human body.

The diagram below gives you an idea of the relative contributions made by the different 'combinations' or compounds to the body of an adult man.

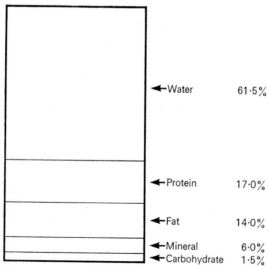

The make-up of man

I have explained what you are in terms of chemicals for one very good reason. I want to show you how chemically similar you are to the food you eat.

The chemical make-up of food

Food is, in simple terms, made up of similar chemical compounds to your own body. Here are a few examples of what I mean:

The make-up of some common food items

Constituents	White bread	Raw beef	Milk	Hard cheese
Water	38%	65%	88%	38%
Protein	8%	18%	3%	25%
Fat	2%	17%	4%	36%
Minerals	less than 0·2%	less than 0.1%	less than 0.1%	1%
Carbohydrate	52%	0%	5%	0%
Total	100%	100%	100%	100%

There are however two main differences between the chemical make-up of yourself and the food you eat.

The first and most obvious one is that the percentages of the different compounds in each food are both different from each other and also from that of your own body. However, it is worth noting that of the four foods listed above, you are most similar in chemical composition to raw beef – which is not altogether surprising since you are mainly flesh and beef is merely the flesh of cattle.

The second difference which is not as obvious is that, for instance, the protein about which I have been talking is not just one protein but many different proteins, and it is the same, although there are not so many alternative kinds for fat and carbohydrate. And the forms that the proteins and fats, but not the carbohydrates, usually adopt inside your own body are different from those in the food you eat. But I shall be telling you more about this in the next section of this chapter when I talk about each of these nutrients in more detail.

However, the water and minerals that are found both in your body and in the food you eat are the same. And there is one further group of substances that I haven't yet mentioned, because they are present in such minute quantities in comparison with all the other compounds, and they are the same both in your body and in the food you eat. These are known as the vitamins and even though they are hardly present they are, as their name implies, vital if you are to continue living healthily, a point upon which I shall be expanding later in the chapter.

So there are basic chemical similarities between yourself and the food you eat but that still doesn't bring you any nearer to being able to answer the question 'Why eat?'

In straightforward terms, you eat because you are alive rather than lifeless; being alive means that you have the ability to grow by building up your body tissue and to keep yourself in tip-top condition by constantly repairing and replacing parts that have become worn out. But this growth and repair process can't take place without the presence of energy. In addition, you need energy for any activity you undertake such as walking or sitting or even breathing. Food not only supplies you with this power to operate, it also furnishes you with the building blocks and spare parts that you need for growth and upkeep.

The analogy of the car

I know it is not a perfect analogy and that you will have to stretch your imagination somewhat, but just compare yourself with a car which started off life as a little two-seater. First of all it needed to be built in a garage in much the same way as you are 'built' within your mother's womb. It is then let loose on the roads and falls into the hands of rather a keen car mechanic who has a liking for 'building-up' little cars. Gradually this two-seater is converted, with the help of many bits and pieces from the garage and a good deal of energy on the part of the car mechanic, into a rather grand four-seater. Such is the pride he has in his achievement that he decides to hold on to his 'new' de-luxe model, keeping it constantly in tip-top condition by replacing worn parts and running it with the help of petrol which supplies the necessary energy.

Of course, the car isn't nearly as 'clever' as you are; it must obtain its supplies of building blocks, repair material and energy from many different sources, but yours come solely from the food you eat. It, too, must have outside help when being built, maintained and run, where you don't need such aid. You have the ability to use your food in the way you need it to be used if you are to carry on living, to break it down into the simplest constituents of the chemical compounds I mentioned earlier and to use those parts accordingly.

To understand just how you do this consider what happens to food once inside your mouth. Eating is something you're so used to doing that I'm sure you very seldom stop to think about it.

Your digestive system

Food can only be of use to your body's conversion (or metabolic) factory if it is reduced to its constituent components and this process is carried out by your digestive system, a small diagram of which is shown below.

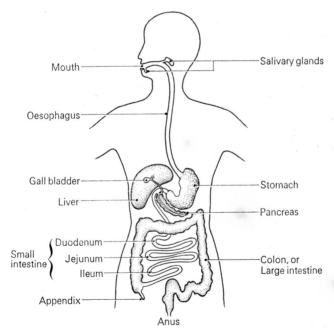

Diagram of the digestive system

In the mouth your food is broken down mechanically by chewing (which underlines the need to have healthy teeth and gums), and it is also automatically mixed with saliva. This substance not only eases the passage of food down the oesophagus to your stomach because it is a rather slimy mixture, but it also starts breaking down the food chemically.

Once in the stomach it is further broken down both chemically and mechanically. From there it passes into the small intestine which, contrary to the implication in its name, is the longest part of your digestive system and is composed of three distinct parts: the duodenum, the jejunum and the ileum. It is here that most of the digestive processes take place; the breakdown chemicals come not only from the wall of the small intestine, but also from the gall bladder and the pancreas. The end result is separated constituents of food — mainly *nutrients* (protein, carbohydrate, fat, vitamins and minerals) — which can now be absorbed into the bloodstream and circulated to those parts of your body which have need of them. (In fact, to be truly precise, a small amount of absorption also takes place in the stomach.) The large intestine is merely part of the waste disposal works, and is the short-term haven for any indigestible items which have travelled through the rest of the system. It is into this part that you would find passing roughage or dietary fibre (which is mostly a very complex carbohydrate); I shall have some words to say about this substance later in this book. From the large intestine the remains are eventually expelled through the anus. This is what happens if all goes well, but it is not always so smooth.

The indigestible facts of digestion

You've no doubt experienced a rather unpleasant pain in the region of your small intestine: probably indigestion. It occurs when items you have been eating are not completely broken down into absorbable substances. It's not always a question of eating too fast; quite frequently it can be caused by being in an emotionally upset state. But whether you are upset or not, absorption of all the totally digested food still takes place.

Now let's take a look at what is absorbed and how each item is used inside your body. So that you don't become too bogged down by constituents of food and thus forget where they originally came from, I shall illustrate this section by imagining that you have just eaten a meal of liver, potato and peas – and for the sake of convenience I shall assume that you ate about 100 g. (3½ oz.) of each of these foods.

The essential role of water

You remember that a large part of you and of the food you eat is made up of water. This meal is no exception: just over half its total weight is water and all of this will be absorbed into your body. Actually, water is the odd one out of all the major absorbable items in food. It is not classed as a nutrient, whereas all the rest are. However, although water is not officially classed as a nutrient it is still essential for life, for without it you would be lucky to last much longer than a week; in comparison, without food you could probably survive for about two months.

You need water for two main reasons: it acts as a stream within which chemicals can easily pass from one part of your body to another and within which chemical changes (or metabolic reactions) can take place, and it keeps the temperature of your body within a very narrow range: this is essential if all the reactions of your body are to proceed as planned.

You lose about two litres (approximately four pints) of water a day but it's not necessary to drink that amount in order to make good your losses. Much of this water comes from the food you eat. As you have just seen about half of the liver, potato and peas is water, and you also obtain a small supply from the reactions which release energy inside your body. So, in fact, you need to drink a good deal less than two litres of fluid a day and in a temperate climate – the one in which you are living – you need only drink when you feel thirsty (in a really hot climate you will need more than this to satisfy the requirements of your body).

The need for nutrients

As I have said, the only other major absorbable items in your diet besides water are the nutrients – the proteins, fats, carbohydrates, minerals and vitamins. The jobs that these substances

undertake within your body fall into three main categories:
energy-givers; body-builders; and protectors.

The energy-givers.   About one-tenth of the liver, potato and
peas would be in the form of carbohydrate and about one-
twentieth would be in the form of fat. The main function of
both these two nutrients is to provide energy, *but* there is a
difference. Carbohydrate is used mainly as a ready source of
energy, whereas fat is used mainly as an energy storage depot
for leaner times. If your energy needs have been satisfied and
you still have spare carbohydrate left over, most of this will be
converted into body fat.

Protein, which like the carbohydrate forms about one-
twentieth of the liver, potato and peas, if it has completed its
prime function of body-building or repairing, can be used as an
energy source and eventually be converted into the energy
storage substance of body fat. So take note: even too much
protein can be fattening.

The need for energy is difficult to understand. Energy is *not*
something you can touch, but it is the power that is required for
you to operate. You are living purely because you are a chemical
process; you are continually changing as a result of millions of
minute chemical reactions which would not proceed without
a supply of energy in the system. In much the same way the car
would not move without a supply of energy which is released
when petrol is burnt in its combustion engine.

Energy is measured in terms of *joules* or *calories*. You're
probably more familiar with the old term of calorie than joule as
it has been well popularized in connection with slimming and
for this reason I shall continue using it throughout the book.

In spite of what I have just told you, you are probably still
confused by calories and carbohydrates, and since it is important
to recognize the difference if ever you try to slim, I feel this is a
point worth labouring.

Let me emphasize: calories are a measure of the *amount* of
energy in food. Carbohydrates are just *one group* of compounds
in food which supply the calories of energy.

Another point on energy: don't think that a well-endowed
food will make you feel that much more active. The decision
to be active comes first, and the energy is used as a result. As I

have already explained, a food which supplies too many calories of energy for your needs is stored as fat, in much the same way as petrol is stored in the car tank. In effect, therefore, too much energy can make you feel less active than just the right amount, because you become overweight and lethargic as a result.

All available energy (i.e. its calorie value) that is provided by the food you eat is eventually lost from your body in the form of heat, so you constantly need a new supply if you are to survive.

The body-builders.   I mentioned above that the prime function of protein is to build up your body and repair it. It is, in fact, the chief nutrient for performing this role. Let me explain why.

You are basically a mass of millions upon millions of tiny, enclosed cells and the walls of each of these are made from protein.

You might think that there is no further need for this nutrient once you are adult and have a complete set of cells but I'm afraid you're wrong if you do. Admittedly, you need less per unit of body weight than when you were actually growing, but you still need some because you are continually losing cells from all parts of your body. For instance, if you have a particularly dry skin you may be more aware of this phenomenon than most. You will, no doubt, have noticed how you must cope with the constant presence of flaky tissue. This is literally a mass of dead cells and will have already been replaced, in the skin beneath, by new tissue needing protein for its formation.

It's really rather like that car I was talking about earlier; when it is being used on the road it is fully grown, if you like, but it is subject to wear and tear and from time to time parts need replacing.

The other main body-building nutrients are the minerals, calcium and phosphorus. These are required for the formation of your bones and your teeth, where you will also find fluorine present in combination as fluoride. This helps make the strong enamel layer. You obviously need a regular supply of these items when you are growing, but you also need some when you are an adult to make up for the continuous loss of skeleton due to wear and tear.

The protectors.   The protectors are found only amongst the minerals and vitamins. They are needed in relatively small amounts just to keep things running smoothly, to 'protect' against upsets, and each is usually found in a wide variety of different foods, the liver, potatoes and peas being no exception.

There are several 'protecting' minerals, but I shall only talk about the ones that affect your diet in a practical kind of way. These are iron and iodine.

Iron is vital for life. It forms an essential part of the red blood pigment haemoglobin which carries oxygen from your lungs to all parts of your body. Without oxygen no energy could be released from the food you eat because chemical reactions just would not take place and you would die. Incidentally, a by-product of these energy-releasing reactions is carbon dioxide which is picked up by your blood, transported to your lungs and expelled in your breath. Hence, the reason for breathing in oxygen and breathing out carbon dioxide.

Despite the fact that a red blood cell only lasts for about 120 days, very little iron is actually lost from your body as a result. You hold on to it in order to make a new cell, so you normally only need a very small supply of iron, once you are fully grown.

Iodine forms part of a group of substances which are to be found in the thyroid gland in your neck. It is these which control the rate of all the chemical reactions in the cells of your body (i.e. they control the rate of metabolism). Hence, the reason why you often hear people blaming their weight problem on an underactive thyroid (which is undoubtedly *not* the reason) – for if the body's chemical reactions proceed at a slower rate than usual then less food will be broken down to provide energy and more will be turned into body fat. A fairly steady supply of iodine is necessary in the diet, as it is regularly lost from your body.

The vitamins

There is almost a whole alphabet of them in number, and I am certainly not going to mention each but will just give you an idea of the main ones and what they do.

First let me briefly illustrate their role in your body by returning to the analogy of the car. There's no doubt it could run without some of the nuts which keep its wheels in place, and the engine, too, would probably operate without one of its sparking plugs, but for how long and how well? The point about vitamins is that you don't need much of them, but they do help you to run smoothly and to last for years.

The jobs performed by the main vitamins are varied. Vitamin A is required for healthy vision and also for the growth of a child.

The B group of vitamins, as they are called, are many in number but you need only worry about three of them: vitamin B1, or thiamin, its chemical name; vitamin B2, or riboflavin, its chemical name; and nicotinic acid. All three of these vitamins help to release calories of energy from the food you eat.

Vitamin C which is the one vitamin you have probably heard about is chemically called ascorbic acid and is needed to form cementing tissue between each body cell and also for absorbing iron into your body.

Finally, you need vitamin D for formation of your bones.

As I have already mentioned, there are many other vitamins, but those described above are the only ones that really concern you in a practical dietary way.

Energy and food constituents – in more detail

I am going to deal with energy first of all since it rather ties this whole section together.

The need for energy

The first point that you must have quite clear in your mind about energy is that it is not something you can touch, rather it is the power that you need to stay alive and to perform different functions.

Energy can be present in several different forms. In the food you eat it is present within the nutrients as chemical energy; it can then be released from your body as heat energy; it can be present in a mechanical form, for example, when you move a boat by means of oars in the water; it can come from the sun; and, finally, it can be in the form of electrical energy.

All forms of energy can be converted into each other without any loss en route. For instance, electrical energy is used to power most modern-day lamps, and if you keep your hand close to a bulb which is on you can feel that it is continually giving off heat because it gets hotter and hotter; the electrical energy is being completely converted into heat energy.

I will now concentrate on the energy in your food.

Inside you

You probably don't know much about chemistry – and maybe you don't want to know too much – but a basic understanding is necessary if you are to come to terms with what is going on inside you.

When food is broken down by your body a good deal of it is burnt with the help of the oxygen from air you breathe in through your lungs to release energy.

This whole process is somewhat similar to the way coal and wood is burnt on a fire. You apply the flame (equivalent to the enzymes, minerals and vitamins – mainly group B – which start the energy-releasing reactions in your body) to the coal and wood (equivalent to the food you eat) which is burnt with the help of oxygen. Ashes remain after the burning process. These are the solid remains – or, in other words, what couldn't be burnt. (Food does contain similar substances, e.g. the minerals. However, it also contains substances – the amino acids to be precise – which if put on a fire would be further broken down releasing heat energy in the process. But, in the body, they are not further broken down. They are built up instead to form proteins which make the walls of the cells. These proteins contain energy and since it is not released it is known as un-available energy.)

Another end product of the burning of wood and coal is the gas, carbon dioxide. Your body cells also produce carbon dioxide when they use oxygen to convert food into energy. This carbon dioxide is carried back to the lungs where it is ex-changed for more oxygen. The carbon dioxide is then breathed out from your lungs.

Water is also given off by the fire in an evaporated form because of the presence of so much heat. (Water, as I have already mentioned, is a by-product of the energy-releasing reactions in your body.)

Finally, a good deal of heat energy is released in the burning process which was the whole reason for lighting the fire in the first place. As I have said before all the available energy from the food you eat is eventually lost as heat and you are continually giving off heat, which is why if it is not too cold – in which case the heat is immediately lost to the surrounding air – your flesh will feel warm.

So much of the food you eat is burnt in a similar way to coal and wood, but that is where the similarity ends. The energy-releasing reactions (involving mainly carbohydrates and fat) inside your body take place in small neat steps which are finely controlled by certain enzymes, minerals and vitamins whereas the burning of coal and wood is one continuous process from beginning to end. But why the need for only small steps? I can only answer this question by taking a look at how the released energy is put to work within your body.

Putting the energy to work

Firstly – and this is where virtually all the energy released ends up – it is used to perform any activities, both involuntary, such as breathing, and voluntary, such as moving your arm or your leg. These involuntary and voluntary activities take place because of the contraction of many muscle fibres. Each contraction needs a small amount of energy which can be supplied by a 'packet of energy' from one of the burning reactions.

Secondly, a very small amount of the released energy is used in the building-up process. Not every reaction in your body results in a breakdown of substances; some make more complicated products, for example, the building blocks of protein – the amino acids (about which I shall be saying something under protein) are rearranged from their plant or original animal form and built up into human protein which is then used to form cell walls – and the building blocks of fat, if they are not needed as a source of immediate energy. Thus although one pound of fat when burnt releases about 3500 Calories of energy, it needs slightly more than this amount to be formed. This building-up process (or synthesis) because it is so complicated, and because so many different substances may be involved, also takes place in a series of many small reactions each of which requires a small 'packet of energy' to proceed.

There is one further point about the synthesis process. To a certain extent the chief nutrients (fat, carbohydrate and protein) can be swopped around. For instance, carbohydrate can readily be turned into fat, and protein can eventually be converted into fat if it has completed its body-building and repairing functions. So you can understand why too much of any type of food will cause you to gain weight in the form of body fat.

Calories and joules

The popular way to measure energy in food is by means of calories.

A calorie with a small 'c' is not a very large amount of energy, and in practice the calorie value of food is actually in terms of kilocalories or Calories with a capital 'C'. A kilocalorie is 1000 times the size of a calorie. But just to confuse matters, wherever the word calorie is used and no specific amount is mentioned then calorie with a small c is used.

In the scientific world energy in food is measured in terms of joules; and very shortly you will be using this term instead of the calorie. Scientists decided, quite sensibly, that since all energy is interchangeable there was little point in having one measure for one form and a completely different measure for another form, so they now use the 'joule', originally just a measure of mechanical energy, for all forms. Actually, it is not so fearsome as it sounds: 4.2 joules are equal to 1 calorie, so in order to get the joule value of a food, say, 25 g. (1 oz.) of bread, you multiply the Calorie value (70) by 4.2 which gives you just over 290 kilojoules. So that you are prepared for the change I have listed both the calorie and the kilojoule value of certain foods in Appendix A on page 155.

Calories in food

The calorie value of food can be worked out in two ways.

Firstly, it can be calculated by drying the food and then totally burning it in oxygen. The amount of heat it gives off as a result of this process can then be converted into the calorie value by deducting the energy contained in the unabsorbed food and in the protein used for body-building and repair. The apparatus for carrying out this procedure is known as the Bomb Calorimeter.

Secondly, it can be calculated by knowing how much of which nutrients are present in the food sample. This is because it is known that 1 g. of pure fat provides about 9 Calories, 1 g. of pure alcohol provides about 7 Calories and finally, 1 g. of both carbohydrate and protein each provide about 4 Calories.

The calories that you need

If you are a male adult then each day you use up approximately 2700 Calories of energy (women use up about 2200). About two-thirds of this is required to just keep you ticking over, for example, to keep your heart and lungs at work, and it is known as your basal metabolic rate (metabolism is the word used to describe all the reactions that take place in your body).

Some people claim that they have an abnormally slow basal metabolic rate (or BMR) and that it is the cause of their weight problem. Their diagnosis is undoubtedly wrong; an abnormally slow BMR is extremely rare and this fact cannot be emphasized too strongly.

The remaining third of your daily calorie expenditure is used up in performing tasks such as sitting, walking or running. The more energetic you are the more calories of energy you use up. For instance when you are sitting down for an hour you only use up about 90 Calories in that time but if you are walking briskly for an hour you may well use up about three times that amount (i.e. 270 Calories). So you see, if you are energetic you do require more calories of energy (and, in practice, that means more to eat) than someone who is rather lazy.

The nutrients whose main job it is to provide these calories of energy are fat and carbohydrate, so let me take a closer look at each of these.

Fat

Fat in the diet is different from fat in the body, and the word is also being used in both these two senses to describe a whole collection of fats.

In food you can both see fats (for instance, butter or fat on meat) and not see them (for instance, the fat in milk and cheese). Fats can also be both solid and liquid (as in oils) at room temperature.

It is important for you to know a little about the chemistry of fats (don't worry, I shall not dwell on it for too long!) because you will find it helps in understanding the chapter on coronary heart disease.

Fats in the diet are basically alike because they are all made from similar building blocks – glycerol and three fatty acids which combine to form triglycerides or neutral fats, as they can be known. Glycerol is more commonly known as glycerine and is a sweet, slightly thick, colourless liquid. It is in the same form in any fat. The three fatty acids, however, vary from fat to fat, and it is these which largely decide what kind of fat it is.

Fatty acids come in three main forms: polyunsaturated, monounsaturated and saturated, and fats usually contain a mixture of all three. But the fats which contain an abnormally large amount of polyunsaturated fatty acids tend to be oils, and vice versa for those containing a good deal of saturated fatty acids.

Fat in your body is merely a collection of triglycerides like the fats in the food you eat, but the two do differ because their triglyceride make-up, due to dissimilar fatty acids, is not the same.

Body fat is stored immediately beneath your skin, but you can also find it around your internal organs, such as the heart, and in the cells of your body. You need a certain amount of body fat, mainly because it keeps you warm but, of course, too much is a bad thing. It throws your whole body off balance.

Body fat does provide protection and warmth and is an excellent way to store calories of energy, but as you know it can be made from carbohydrate and indirectly from protein, so do you, in fact, need to eat fat in the diet, particularly as most of us seem to be suffering from an overabundance of body fat?

Is dietary fat necessary?

One of the most important reasons why you eat fat – and I know you might say that it is the cause of your weight problem – is because it makes your food taste good. Just think how much nicer those boiled potatoes are with a slab of butter on top of them. If you had virtually no fat in your diet your food, I would think, would be so unappetizing as to put you off it for life. So, although perhaps you might not want to make your food taste too good, you do want it to be reasonable.

Dietary fat, from the nutrient point of view, apart from being a good source of calories of energy does provide your body with three essential fatty acids. These are known as essential because they are needed by your body and yet cannot be made by it, even if it is supplied with the required raw materials. Fats also 'carry' with them, and are the chief source of, a few vitamins — the main ones being A and D. And since these nutrients are essential for health, fats must be eaten so that they can be supplied.

Although you do need some fat in your diet it doesn't mean that you should overload your menu with this nutrient. We would probably all be a lot better off if we reduced the amount of fat we ate.

Carbohydrate

Carbohydrate in the diet is the other main source of calories of energy. It is, as you have already seen, a ready source — it can be easily broken down by the cells of your body — whereas fat is more of a storage depot for energy.

'Carbohydrate', like 'fat', is a term used to describe a whole collection of carbohydrates, the most common dietary ones of which are starch and sugar. Starch is chemically much more complicated than sugar and is found in such foods as potatoes, bread, biscuits and cakes. Sugar as you know it is really called sucrose and is just one of about six sugars which are very simple carbohydrates. Three of these form the basic building blocks (not sucrose) of all the other carbohydrates, the other three are each made up of two basic building blocks.

When carbohydrate is digested it is broken down into the three simplest sugars and most of it ends up as glucose, which is one of these sugars, in the blood. This is then either broken down to release energy, put into storage as a complex carbohydrate, glycogen, or converted into fat once the stores of glycogen are full up.

The simplest sugar – glucose

There are two things I would like to say about glucose.

If you are feeling rather tired or low you are sometimes advised by well meaning friends to take glucose (or perhaps you know them as dextrose) tablets to perk you up a bit. However, although glucose is the last link in the breakdown of carbohydrate to release energy, it must have a reason for being broken down, i.e. you must have been active and therefore required the release of energy. If you do not require the energy, glucose, like any other carbohydrate, will mostly be turned into fat.

The second point I would like to make about glucose is this. Normally you have a certain amount of it present in your body, but when you eat some food the level of glucose rises and immediately your body sets about getting it back to normal. In so doing it usually overshoots the mark, particularly if the glucose levels were really raised, and then corrects itself. This is why you may well experience a slight feeling of hunger a short time after a large meal particularly if it was high in carbohydrates, in which case your blood glucose levels will have been greatly raised.

Do you need carbohydrate?

I asked in the previous section whether fat was necessary in your diet, since carbohydrate could equally (and indeed often does) perform fat's function of providing calories of energy, but you saw that fat does a few other rather useful jobs as well and therefore can't be completely excluded. I will now reverse the situation and see if you could do without any carbohydrate in your diet, thus letting fats do all the energy providing work.

On palatability grounds, I'd have to say no to this. A diet without carbohydrate would be pretty well intolerable: no fruit, bread, potatoes, cake, biscuits, buns. It's true that you shouldn't overdo most of them, but to exclude them entirely would be a shame.

There is also another reason why you should at least include some carbohydrate in your diet, and that is because you would suffer from an unpleasant condition known as ketosis if you didn't. Ketosis occurs whenever you use far more fat than carbohydrate as a source of energy. Under these circumstances not all the fat will be completely burnt to carbon dioxide and water as in the normal course of events, but instead it will be broken down to eventually give a substance known as acetone (and if you don't know what that is, just smell the contents of a bottle of nail varnish — you soon will!). So even a small amount of carbohydrate is necessary in your diet.

Cellulose

I must not leave carbohydrate without mentioning a very complicated one which is not broken down by your digestive system and therefore not absorbed. It is called cellulose, and together with a few bits and pieces of vegetable matter, it forms what you know as roughage or dietary fibre. For many years this was thought to be just a waste substance, but more recently it has been named by some as the cure for all ills. I look at it and its sources slightly more closely in Chapter 6.

Now there is one other nutrient which supplies calories of energy, but its main job is to build up your body and it is known as protein.

Protein

'Protein' like 'carbohydrate' and 'fat' is a collective name for many different proteins and these are formed from a group of just twenty basic building blocks or amino acids.

All proteins from the food you eat are broken down by your digestive system into amino acids before they are absorbed into your body. They are then rebuilt into proteins which are uniquely yours and which are distinctly different from those of other animals or vegetables.

Proteins are mainly used to build the walls of all your cells, but they are also found as enzymes, which spark off many of the reactions of your body, and as antibodies, which fight any uninvited substances and, in consequence, protect you from disease.

You need protein in your diet even if you have stopped growing — although your needs won't be so great at this time —

because your cells are continually being broken down and lost and therefore new ones must be formed which require protein for their formation.

Essential amino acids

Twelve of the twenty amino acids which are used to form your protein can be made by your own body if the basic ingredients (carbon and nitrogen) are available, but the remaining eight must be supplied ready-made by your diet (two more are needed if you are actively growing). These eight amino acids are known as the essential amino acids.

Which protein is best?

You might have heard people saying that protein from one source is not as good for you as protein from another source. What truth is there in such a statement?

Well, there is something to be said for it, and it's all due to those eight amino acids that are so essential for your body.

A protein is a very large substance (molecule to be precise) composed of many, many amino acids, and for its formation it needs just the right amount of amino acids to be present. Of course, the ones that your body can make are no problem, but the ones it can't – the essential amino acids – must be present in just the right amounts in order for the protein to be made. If even one is slightly lacking then *none* of the protein can be formed.

The proteins found in other animals tend to be made in a more similar way to yours than those found in vegetables, i.e. they have more of the essential amino acids present in the required amounts. Thus you can make better use of the animal proteins than the vegetable ones. Any amino acids which cannot be used to form protein are broken down to release calories of energy or are converted into the carbohydrate, glucose and thence to body fat.

But do not now think that vegetables proteins are a complete waste of time. They can provide a valuable addition to the amino acids from animal proteins; after all, even though their selection of essential amino acids is not quite what is needed by your body, they do still provide some, and these can always be used to supplement those that may be lacking from an animal source, or, indeed, as vegetarians would be quick to point out, combinations of vegetable proteins, such as those from flour and pulses, can provide a very useful selection of essential amino acids.

That completes protein and so at this stage I am going to turn to the lesser mortals in your diet. I have discussed the three main nutrients, now let me take a peep at the minerals and the vitamins which, in terms of weight, form a much, much smaller part of you and of your diet. I shall look firstly at the minerals.

The minerals

Virtually all the minerals known to man can be found in your body. However, only about fifteen are actually of use and therefore must be supplied by the diet.

Some of these essential items are more necessary than others, and I shall take a look at only the very important ones starting with the three needed for healthy bone and teeth formation.

Calcium. This is the most plentiful mineral in your body; it combines both with phosphorus and with one or two other substances to form the hard cementing substance of bone which is found between another substance: cartilage, a protein, which is relatively soft. Contrary to popular belief nails and hair, the other two hard parts of your body, contain very little calcium and phosphorus. They are largely made of protein called keratin, and thus however much you eat of a calcium or phosphorus rich food it won't make your split ends or your cracked nails any better; neither are in that state because of lack of calcium or phosphorus.

Like the cells of your body, calcium and phosphorus are continually being removed and therefore they must be replaced. So even though you need a particularly large amount, especially of calcium, when you are actively growing, you still need some when you have stopped increasing in size.

So far I have just talked about the role that calcium and phosphorus play in the bones and teeth and indeed this is their most important function, but they do carry out other jobs.

Calcium is needed for the blood-clotting process; for

B

instance, even the slightest scratch would be a major problem without the presence of calcium. It is also needed for the process of sending messages from your brain along your nerves and to keep your muscles in a ready-for-action state.

Phosphorus.   This mineral is needed for even more jobs than calcium. It is an essential part of the life and work of each of your cells, and it also helps some of the B vitamins – the ones that spark off the energy-releasing reactions – to carry out their work.

Phosphorus is present in such a wide variety of foods that you have no need to worry about getting enough. Calcium, however, is slightly different because its sources are a bit limited in number (I shall be looking at them near the end of this chapter). There is another problem with this mineral: your body does not let it in too easily; only about twenty to fifty per cent is absorbed, and the rest passes straight through your digestive system and out. This figure is affected by several different factors:

1   You will absorb more if you have only eaten a small amount of it and vice versa if you have taken in a particularly large amount.
2   Vitamin D is needed for the absorption process, and if this is lacking less calcium will be taken in.
3   There is a substance found in bran (the outer part of a wheat grain), nuts and pulses called phytic acid which combines with calcium and prevents it from being absorbed. But this acid is to some extent prevented from doing its unwanted work on calcium in the presence of yeast. Thus, the calcium in wholemeal bread, which contains plenty of yeast, is not too badly affected by the phytic acid which is found in the branny part of this bread.
4   Oxalic acid, found in such foods as spinach, rhubarb and strawberries, works in a similar way to phytic acid, but since these foods do not form a very large part of your diet this interference is not really worth worrying about.
5   Finally, absorption of calcium is affected by Glauber's and Epsom salts.

But on a good note, absorption of calcium is increased in the presence of protein, fruit and vegetables. Thus foods which contain both calcium and protein, such as milk and products made from milk, are particularly useful sources of calcium and so are dishes combining milk and fruit or vegetables.

Actually, in this country we don't need to worry too much about lack of calcium because we all eat a fair amount of the calcium-rich foods; the difficulties of absorption just present those people who have to decide how much we actually need with a bit of a headache!

Fluorine. A final brief word must be given to fluorine before I leave this group. It is found in the hard, outer coating of your teeth — the enamel — in the form of fluoride and it has been shown to protect them against dental decay, particularly so in the teeth of young children.

Fluoride is mainly supplied by the water you drink, and this is the reason why it is added to this substance. There is absolutely no danger to health in doing this, so long as it is properly controlled, but you may not like the idea of being forced to take a substance you don't in fact need (because you don't happen to have dental decay). Certainly there is something to be said for this view and perhaps it would be a good idea if just those individuals — the children — who really are at risk for developing decay should take a supplement of fluoride. It could possibly be added to certain sweets which they particularly like, but this form of supplementation must never let mums think that all will be well with their children's teeth. Children must still be encouraged to brush their teeth regularly and to cut down on the sticky buns between meals.

Iron. About half the iron in your body forms part of the complex substance known as haemoglobin, which is found in your red blood cells and performs the very important tasks of, firstly, carrying oxygen to all the cells of your body, so that they can then break down the energy-containing nutrients from your diet and, secondly, carrying one of the waste products of these reactions — carbon dioxide — back to your lungs so that it can be got rid of in the air you breathe out.

The other half of your body iron is not found in the red blood cells but in the other cells of your body, and this iron is closely connected with the release of oxygen from the haemoglobin in readiness for the energy-releasing reactions.

The red blood cells are continually being broken down together with the haemoglobin they contain, and the iron instead of being lost from the body is mostly kept for the formation of new red blood cells. So, in the normal course of events you don't need that much iron in your diet, but, if you suddenly lose a great amount of blood, such as during a haemorrhage or, for women, during menstruation, you will need to replace that which you have lost. This is the reason why it is more important for a menstruating woman to have the extra portion of red meat (which is rich in iron) than the men.

Lack of iron in the diet is quite common even in this country, and one of the main reasons why is that only between five to twenty per cent of dietary iron is absorbed by your body. There are several reasons for this: 1) As with calcium, iron absorption is lessened by the presence of phytic acid (found in bran, nuts and pulses) and oxalic acid (found in spinach, rhubarb and strawberries); there are other foods but these are the ones most likely to be included in your diet; 2) some iron is not available for absorption until it has been worked upon by hydrochloric acid, which is found in your stomach. Certain people have a particularly low amount of this substance in their stomach and therefore their dietary iron is not well absorbed; 3) lack of vitamin C will cause decreased absorption and therefore it's always a good idea to eat iron and vitamin C-rich foods together — such a combination would be red meat and fresh vegetables; 4) and, finally, iron from vegetables seems to be very much less easily absorbed than iron from animals, although we don't quite know why.

If you are particularly short of iron you will absorb more than you need, and vice versa if you have plenty, thus recommending how much iron you should take is a difficult task.

Sodium and Potassium.   I don't propose to say much about these two minerals because you have more than enough of them in the diet you eat. However, it is worth making the point that people who sweat a lot do need more sodium than people who don't sweat much, because a good deal of this mineral is lost in this way. This does not apply to potassium.

Both of these minerals are needed chiefly to control the amount of water you have in your body, and if taken in excessive amounts, they are passed out of your body. However, this process is totally dependent upon your kidneys. If these aren't functioning properly which only happens when you are rather ill, *not* when you are just overweight, you will hold on to too much and, in consequence, become bloated with water. But, let me emphasize, this only happens when you are ill, not when you are overweight, so there is no real point in taking pills known as diuretics to get rid of what you think is the chief cause of your weight problem — excess water. What you really need to do is to get rid of your excess fat.

The kidneys of very young children aren't able to cope with too much sodium (in the form of salt) and therefore it is important that you don't add salt to their food. Apart from anything else they don't like salty food in the same way as you do. (Recently there was a bit of an outcry about a yeast-extract product, which is particularly salty, being recommended for babies.)

Iodine. This mineral is used to form a mixture of hormones (substances which switch the organs of your body into action) found in the thyroid gland in your neck. These are very important because they control the rate at which all the reactions of your body (the rate of metabolism) will take place. However, as with the other minerals, enough is as good as a feast; your body will not suddenly speed up and break down extra fat to release energy as is implied by some manufacturers who sell iodine-rich products to help you slim.

A lack of iodine is not common in this country these days, although it used to be. Some plants, especially cabbage and related vegetables, interfere with the thyroid hormone and thus cause your requirements for iodine to be increased, but I wouldn't therefore recommend that you cut down your intake of cabbage. If there is a possibility of shortage it is much more sensible to increase your intake of iodine-rich foods, such as salt which has had iodine added to it, or fish.

The vitamins

These are substances which can't be made by your body and therefore must be included in your diet. They are only needed in very, very small amounts, but they are vital for keeping you really healthy. If you don't eat enough of them then eventually you will suffer from very definite diseases, and I shall outline these in the next section of this chapter.

Vitamins can either be soluble in water, in which case there is no danger of eating too much, or soluble in fat, in which case there can be danger in eating too much because excess can't easily be disposed of by your body's water-works.

Some vitamins have more practical importance to you than others, and I only propose to look at those about which you might need to worry.

Vitamin A.   This is needed mainly for seeing in dim light; it forms part of a pigment in your eye which is found in the cells of your retina: the layer at the back of your eyeball which picks up light. Vitamin A is also needed for child growth and protection against infections.

If you read a list of ingredients on a packet or tin of food which tells you not only which nutrients are present but also how much there is of each, you will see that the quantity of vitamin A is recorded in retinol equivalents. This is because vitamin A is chemically present in food in two different forms, retinol being one of them. To make life easier all vitamin A is measured in terms of retinol, even if it is not in fact retinol, hence the term retinol equivalents.

Vitamin A is fat soluble, and it is largely found in fatty food, although not always. In order for it to be absorbed into your body there must be some fat present, thus even if you are eating a good deal of the vitamin but having only very little fat, you are nevertheless likely to be deficient. However, as it is fat soluble and you can therefore store it in your body, you will only show signs of a lack when this store is nearly used up.

Vitamins of the B group.   These, although all chemically very different, do have certain points in common. They are all soluble in water and thus the body doesn't store them, so there is no danger of excess. There can be a danger of too little, although it's very unlikely to happen in this country. They also all work together with the enzymes of your body: the substances which spark off many of the chemical reactions.

There are just three that I am going to talk about. These are the main ones, and they all help to release calories of energy from the food you eat.

Vitamin B1, or thiamin, is needed for the continuous release of calories of energy from carbohydrates, and thus the amount that you require is dependent upon how much carbohydrate you eat. So, in fact, we in this country, who eat less carbohydrate than those of the underdeveloped world, likewise need less vitamin B1 than they do (in fact, we usually end up eating a good deal more).

One other point about this vitamin is that it is very easily destroyed by heat, particularly in alkaline conditions such as occurs with sodium bicarbonate in water.

Vitamin B2, or riboflavin, also helps to release calories of energy from carbohydrate, and therefore, the quantities needed are dependent upon the amount of carbohydrate eaten.

Nicotinic acid has one or two other names which you may have come across; for instance, it is known as niacin in the United States. (The latter name may be better because there is a danger of getting nicotinic acid muddled up with nicotine with which it has absolutely *nothing* in common.) As with the two other B vitamins, it helps to release energy from carbohydrate. If you eat a good deal of maize you will either need to eat slightly more nicotinic acid than usual because much of it is unavailable for absorption in maize, or you will need to soak the maize overnight in limewater, which releases the nicotinic acid from its bound form.

Vitamin C.   Chemically known as ascorbic acid, this is, perhaps, the most well known of all the vitamins, largely because of its possible link with curing the common cold. You probably also know that a lack of it eventually causes scurvy, a disease which was common amongst sailors before the present century because fruit and vegetables (the two riches sources of this vitamin) were hard to come by while at sea for long periods of time.

Vitamin C is needed mainly to keep your connective tissue healthy, thus if there is a lack of it you start letting blood through and, in particular, your gums begin to bleed. Similarly wounds take some time longer to heal than usual, because the connective tissue can't immediately be formed.

Vitamin C, as I have already pointed out, also helps you to absorb iron, so it's a good idea to eat vitamin C and iron-rich foods together.

It is water soluble and therefore you need a regular supply because it is not stored by the body to any great extent. It is also the one nutrient which can be very easily lost from food, if the latter is not properly handled. For example, it is very easily changed in the presence of oxygen (which in practice means air), so don't leave cut surfaces of vitamin C-rich foods around for too long; it is also changed by heat, so overcooking will have a drastic effect on this nutrient.

The evidence that excessive amounts of vitamin C intake will protect you from and even cure the common cold is thin, and you would probably be well advised to just forget about the whole business; I might add that this advice includes both vitamin C and the common cold. After all, there is no more effective cure for an illness than forgetting that you are even unwell.

Vitamin D.   This is mainly needed for the absorption of calcium into the body, so if it is lacking it can cause a shortage of calcium in your body, even though this mineral may not be lacking from your diet.

It is fat soluble and therefore can be stored by your body, but, in consequence, there is a danger of overdoing it, which shows itself as an excess absorption of calcium.

Vitamin D shortage sometimes occurs in this country because it is only found in large amounts in a very few foods (which I shall tell you about in the final section of this chapter). It can also be made when your body is exposed to sunlight. Thus people who don't go out often, or who always remain well covered when they go out and who don't eat many vitamin D-rich foods are likely to be at risk. These conditions apply mainly to the elderly.

And with that I have come to the end of the section about the functions of energy and nutrients, so now let me move on to the question of quantity and the effects of not getting the right amount.

How much and too much or too little

From what I have told you so far you must realize that you need a pretty regular supply of all the nutrients in certain quantities to be completely healthy.

Tables have been drawn up by the governments of most countries (the ones for this country are shown in Appendix B on page 172) which give recommended quantities of energy and the nutrient intakes for people of all ages. However, these do differ from country to country, mainly because the kinds of foods normally eaten vary and thus the recommendations must be altered accordingly, and also because it is very difficult to be really precise about what is needed and not every government reaches the same conclusion.

How are the recommendations calculated?

First of all it must be decided what the aim of the recommendations should be. After all, good nutrition for a pig, which will eventually supply pork meat and thus be must well fattened, is not really what you are after — although you might think so when you take a look at an average collection of people in this country. What you want is a healthy, which means free from disease, and prolonged life. It really is a bit vague isn't it? Perhaps a little more helpful is a reasonably fast rate of growth. This is usually assumed to go hand in hand with a good diet and vice versa for a poor growth rate.

With these points in mind the people responsible for recommending intakes set about their task of finding out how much is needed by each age group, and I shall look first of all at the nutrients and then at energy because it needs to be treated in a slightly different fashion.

Nutrient needs

If you are short of any nutrients you will eventually develop specific symptoms, but between true health and actual disease is a hazy area in which you are not really on peak form and are, therefore, more likely to become ill. As you might imagine, this hazy area makes it extremely difficult for anyone to reach conclusions about what is really needed.

Despite the problems involved, recommendations must still be found, because they are a useful guideline for those who must plan meals on a large scale and also for doctors who must diagnose an illness from rather vague symptoms, which may be due to lack of a particular nutrient.

In the search for nutrient recommendations, there are three main plans of attack. The first and oldest method is to take a look at different populations of people, see which ones show signs of deficiency and which ones don't, work out how much (not an easy job) of the specific nutrient, on average, each is eating and from these figures calculate a requirement. As you might imagine this method, at best, could only be said to give a rough guide.

The second method is carried out on other animals. They are fed diets containing different amounts of the nutrient under study and that quantity which produces a healthy animal – a somewhat difficult conclusion to draw – is considered to be the best amount. There is then the problem of altering this amount to that required by you or me – this can only ever be an approximate calculation.

The same kind of study can be carried out on human beings, but the practical problems involved – for instance, getting volunteers to participate in the experiment in the first place and also getting them to keep to the test diet – are enormous. Also, as with other animals there is always the difficulty of knowing when a person has reached his most healthy state.

The third and final plan of attack is to carry out balance studies and saturation tests on human beings.

These both work on the assumption that if you have enough of a certain nutrient – and these tests can only apply to those nutrients which can easily be got rid of by your water-works, i.e. not those that are soluble in fat – then you excrete it in an amount that is exactly equal to the quantity you have eaten, i.e. you are in balance for this nutrient and your tissues are saturated with it. However, there are people who disagree with this assumption. They feel that you need to be more than just in balance to achieve real health.

So you can see the problems involved in determining the best dose of a nutrient for the average person are enormous. Note that I say average; there is a *considerable* amount of variation from one person to another which can also be affected by what else they are eating and if they are ill or not, so when a recommendation is eventually arrived at these facts must be taken into consideration as well. Therefore, the figures given in the table in the appendix are about fifty per cent above the average requirement and should cover the needs of about ninety five per cent of the population. So it is very important for you to realize that even though you might be eating less of a certain nutrient than is recommended you will not necessarily be going short.

Energy needs

Energy needs are easier to determine but again there is the problem of individual variation, so you must always remember that the figures given in the back of this book are only average.

Your need for energy is directly related to how much you lose from your body, and this can be fairly accurately measured. It is largely dependent upon how big you are, and thus if you are overweight you would appear to need more energy than if you are at your correct weight. But, as many doctors frequently ask, what is correct weight? Presumably it is the weight at which a person is most healthy. Thus we face the same problem as we did for working out requirements for nutrients: we don't know when a person is really healthy.

To a certain extent you can adapt to more or less energy intake. Some people are better at doing this than others, which may help to explain why some people get fat so easily, but it is important, much more so than with nutrients, that you keep your intake within certain limits or else !

At this point it is perhaps a good idea for me to look at what occurs if that 'or else' should ever happen to you and in this next section I shall consider not only energy, but also all the nutrients which I have just been talking about.

Over and under the required amount

I think the best way of tackling this is to put all the information down in the form of a table and to indicate which of the

The effects of too much or too little

	Too much	Is it likely to happen in Great Britain?	Too little	Is it likely to happen in Great Britain?
Energy	Become fat.	Yes, it is all too common.	Become thin and, in extreme starvation, children develop a disease called marasmus.	Unlikely unless it is done deliberately.
The Nutrients				
Protein	Can be used as a source of calories.	Yes. We eat more than enough protein and some of it is used as a calorie source.	In extreme cases children develop a disease called kwashiorkor.	No.
Calcium	Virtually unknown.	—	A disease called rickets occurs in children; in adult women, who have had many pregnancies, a disease called osteomalacia may occur; and in the elderly a disease	Rickets and osteomalacia are very unlikely; osteoporosis can occur amongst elderly people but the cause may well not be a dietary one. At present it is not known.

called osteoporosis may occur. All three diseases affect the bones.

Phosphorus	Cannot occur.		Unknown because phosphorus occurs in so many different foods.	—
Fluorine	Gives brown mottling of the teeth.	Very unlikely.	Not certain whether it is essential, but it can help prevent tooth decay.	Tooth decay can be somewhat prevented with more fluorine.
Iron	Not possible.	—	This is the commonest cause of anaemia.	Some women suffer from mild forms of this disease.
Sodium	Leads to fluid retention; but this is normally due to the kidneys not working properly. Babies can have too much.	Both are possible but neither is common.	Muscle cramps, apathy, loss of weight, and, perhaps, being sick.	Not likely (it only happens in really hot climates).

	Too much	Is it likely to happen in Great Britain?	Too little	Is it likely to happen in Great Britain?
Potassium	Not possible.	—	Not possible under normal circumstances because potassium in the diet is so wide-spread.	No.
Iodine	Not possible.	—	A goitre develops which is an enlargement of the thyroid gland and usually means there is slight lack of iodine. There are more extreme signs of deficiency.	Slight goitre does exist to a very small extent in this country.
Vitamin A	A great deal too much can be poisonous.	Does occasionally occur; it is most likely in children, but there is one well-reported case of a health-food nut who poisoned himself with this substance.	Results in night blindness.	No.

Vitamin				
Vitamin B1	Not possible.	—	Eventually the deficiency disease beri-beri results.	No.
Vitamin B2	Not possible.	—	Eventually sores appear on the lips, tongue and skin.	No.
Nicotinic Acid	Not possible.	—	Eventually the disease called pellagra results.	No.
Vitamin C	Perhaps very large doses cure the common cold, but it is very unlikely.	—	Eventually the deficiency disease called scurvy results.	Sometimes occurs amongst old people and bachelors who are cooking for themselves.
Vitamin D	Causes excess absorption of calcium; young children are especially likely to be hit.	Occasionally it happens.	The same as for calcium.	The same as for calcium.

complaints, if any, are likely to affect you or any member of your family who is living in Britain or, indeed in any western country, today.

Foods which supply useful amounts of the main nutrients

Nutrient	Food
Protein	meat, fish, eggs, cheese, milk, bread, nuts, beans, peas
Carbohydrate	sugar, bread, cakes, biscuits, sweets, potatoes, pastry
Fat	butter, margarine, cooking oil, cream, cheese, salad dressing
Calcium	milk, cheese, bread, fish eaten with bones e.g. sardines
Iodine	iodized salt, fish
Iron	offal meat, red meat, egg yolk, bread, curry and cocoa powder, sardines, dried prunes and apricots, oatmeal, treacle, pulses
Vitamin A	fish liver oil, margarine, butter, carrots, liver , hard cheese
B group:	
(Vitamin B1 – Thiamin)	yeast, pork, peas, bread, cod's roe, bacon, oatmeal, liver, kidneys, flour (including enriched white and soya), peanuts and brazil nuts, wheatgerm
(Vitamin B2 – Riboflavin)	yeast, liver, hard cheese, milk. liver, kidney, egg, almonds
(Nicotinic Acid)	yeast, liver, beef, fish, peas, bread, all meats. peanuts, pulses, soya flour, beer, barley
Vitamin C	green vegetables, fresh citrus fruits, potatoes
Vitamin D	cod liver oil, oily fish, margarine, eggs, butter, liver, cod's roe.

(Note: I have excluded phosphorus and potassium from this list because they are present in so many foods, and also sodium which is richly present in salt).

There is a sure and certain way to avoid repercussions of too much or too little and that is by eating a properly balanced diet, which brings me on to the last section of this chapter.

How to achieve a well-balanced diet

It's all too easy to get totally carried away with the separate nutrients and with energy and forget that what *you* want to know about is the food you must eat, which is nearly always a collection of nutrients. Quite often one nutrient or maybe two or three will be more plentiful than others, so it is worth your while, for practical purposes and so that you are not misled by any advertisements, to know which foods are good sources of which nutrients. The table on page 48 should help you with this, and so should the table in Appendix A where I have outlined which of the common foods are good sources of what.

So that you can be sure of a well-balanced diet, which means that you will be getting all the nutrients you need in the right amounts, you don't have to follow one strict monotonous menu; if you choose foods from as many different sources (within reason) as possible you can be pretty certain that you are really getting all you need. But just to keep you 'within reason' I have provided some simple guidelines:

1   You should try to have three meals a day, two of which you can class as main and avoid, if possible, any in-between meal eating.
2   The basis of each of your meals should be a food which is rich in protein, so take a look at the table on page 48 to remind yourself what you should be eating.
3   Plenty of fruit and vegetables are always a good idea but make a point of including them in your two main meals at least.
4   Finally, those old high-calorie foods, the ones rich in fat and carbohydrate, must be given a mention. You certainly need some, particularly the fatty ones which also provide vitamins A and D, but, if you can help it, *don't overdo them*.

It's boring to have rules — because that is really what these are — I know, but try not to think of them in that light but, rather, as your passport to a healthy and happy life.

2 The diet of the adult

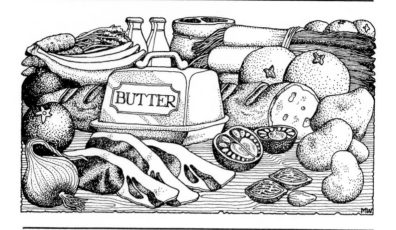

Growth is completed and you are leading a life-style which probably won't change much over thirty to forty years. In consequence the nutritional requirements of your body will remain pretty much the same. But the problem is: 'What should you eat in order to satisfy them?' For instance, do you need what some people like to call a 'proper' breakfast of bacon, sausage, fried egg, tomato and lashings of hot buttered toast and, if not, what should you be having first thing?

Before I supply an answer to the above question just turn your thoughts a moment to the nutritional recommendations for a balanced diet that are given in full on page 51.

The trouble with putting requirements in terms of figures is that everything is made to seem so precise, which in reality is not the case as pointed out in the first chapter. If your weekly diet provides, on average, somewhere in the region of the recommendations opposite (the only one you need to be fairly precise with is energy), then you can be certain that you are eating what you need. The kind of diet that will do this for you, because I realize you have no means of translating what you eat into nutrients and energy, is one which follows the rules I laid down on page 49. To prove the point I have devised a typical

Daily nutritional recommendations of an average adult man or woman leading a sedentary life

The requirements	Man		Woman
	18–35	36–65	18–55
Energy (Calories)	2700	2600	2200
Nutrients			
Protein (g.)	68	65	55
Vitamin B1 (mg)	1.1	1.0	0.9
Vitamin B2 (mg)		1.7	1.3
Nicotinic acid equivalent (mg)		18	15
Vitamin C (mg)		30	30
Vitamin A (retinol equivalent) (μg)		750	750
Vitamin D (μg)		2.5	2.5
Calcium (mg)		500	500
Iron (mg)		10	12

Source: D H S S 1969

menu which is outlined below and on pages 52/53 I show you just what it provides in terms of energy and nutrients. The chart, although a little complicated at first sight, does serve a very useful purpose when it comes to explaining the points about diet which often worry people.

Typical menu for an adult woman

Breakfast	Poached egg on toast
	Toast and marmalade
	Coffee with milk
Mid-Morning	Coffee with milk
Lunch	Baked beans on toast with two grilled sausages and a tomato
	An orange
	Coffee with milk
Mid-Afternoon	Tea with milk
Dinner	Pork chop with green beans, potatoes and gravy
	Fresh fruit salad and ice cream
	Coffee with milk
Bed-Time	Milky coffee

Energy and nutrient breakdown of the typical menu

Food		Energy (Calories)	Protein (gm)	Thiamin (mg)	Riboflavin (mg)	Nicotinic Acid Equivalent (mg)	Vitamin C (mg)	Vitamin A retinol equivalent (µg)	Vitamin D (µg)	Calcium (mg)	Iron (mg)
Breakfast											
Egg	(2 oz)	80	6.8	0.06	0.2	1.8	–	170	0.86	32	1.4
Bread	(1½ oz)	105	3.6	0.075	–	1.05	–	–	–	42	0.75
Margarine	(½ oz)	110	0.05	–	–	–	–	127.5	1.14	0.5	0.05
Marmalade	(1 oz)	35	–	–	–	–	3	2	–	10	0.2
Bread	(1½ oz)	105	3.6	0.075	–	1.05	–	–	–	42	0.75
Margarine	(½ oz)	110	0.05	–	–	–	–	127.5	1.14	0.5	0.05
Milk	(1 oz)	20	0.9	0.01	0.04	0.3	1	12	0.01	34	–
Total		565	15	0.22	0.24	4.2	4	439	3.15	161	3.2
Lunch											
Baked Beans	(5 oz)	120	8.5	0.1	0.5	2.0	5	70	–	90	3
Sausages	(4 oz)	265	11.6	0.92	0.24	10.4	–	–	–	8	2.8
Tomato	(2 oz)	10	0.6	0.04	0.02	0.4	12	66	–	8	0.2
Bread	(1½ oz)	105	3.6	0.075	–	1.05	–	–	–	42	0.75
Margarine	(½ oz)	110	0.05	0.12	–	–	–	127.5	1.14	0.5	0.05
Orange	(4 oz)	40	0.8	0.12	0.04	0.04	56	8	–	48	0.4
Milk	(1 oz)	20	0.9	0.01	0.04	0.3	1	12	0.01	34	–
Total		670	26.05	1.26	0.84	14.2	74	283.5	1.15	230.5	7.2

Dinner										
Grilled Pork Chop (5 oz)	300	17	0.55	0.3	8.5	—	—	—	25	1.5
Green Beans (5 oz)	10	1.5	0.05	0.15	2.0	30	70	—	45	1.0
Boiled Potatoes (5 oz)	160	2.0	0.1	0.05	1.5	10	—	—	5	0.5
Gravy (2 tbls)	60		Negligible	Negligible	Contribution			—		
Fruit Salad (5 oz)	120	1.0	0.1	0.05	0.5	30	20	—	20	0.5
Ice Cream (2 oz)	100	2.4	Negligible	Negligible	Contribution			—	77.8	0.16
Milk (1 oz)	20	0.9	0.01	0.04	0.3	1	12	0.01	34	—
Total	770	24.8	0.067	0.27	2.01	8.7	80.4	0.067	206.8	3.66
Extras										
Milk (9 fl oz)	125	7.83	0.087	0.35	2.61	8.7	104.4	0.087	295.8	—
Grand total	2175	73.68	2.4	2.02	33.8	157.7	928.9	4.4	794.1	14.06
Recommendations										
For Women	2200	55	0.9	1.3	15	30	750	2.5	500	12
For Men	2600–2700	65–68	1.0–1.1	1.7	18	30	750	2.5	500	10

Men's diets versus women's diets

Is it important for him, for instance, to have that extra piece of meat? If you take a close look at the nutrients and energy provided by the diet above and compare them with a man's requirements you can see that all except the energy recommendation are more than adequately met. No special need to eat the meat for that! A few extra potatoes and bread or a couple of pints of beer at the local are all that is wanted. In fact, if I had to make a choice about giving that extra piece of meat to either a man or a woman I would plump for the woman, because her needs for iron, a nutrient which can be lacking in diets, is greater than a man's due to monthly loss in menstruation and meat is a good source of iron.

While on the subject of iron let me look at the importance of liver in a diet. This food is a good source of many nutrients, particularly iron and B vitamins; in consequence at least one portion a week is often recommended by dieticians. Certainly it is good advice to follow if you wish to make sure of a well-balanced intake, but what happens if you literally can't stand the food, which I know is the feeling of quite a few individuals. Can you survive without it? Most certainly, if you are keeping to my rules for a well-balanced diet, and the nutrient breakdown above confirms what I have just said – the iron and B vitamin requirements are more than adequately met *without* the presence of liver in the menu.

Now let me return to that question I posed at the start of this chapter.

Breakfast

A quick analysis shows that the 'proper' breakfast I described would provide about 1300 Calories, or just under half your daily energy requirements. A meal of this size is not such a good idea for breakfast, since it will leave rather a large gap in your allowance for the rest of the day, and in consequence, you will probably end up over-eating. The other point to consider is the over-loading effect. Your body can function more efficiently if the food it receives is evenly spaced throughout the day; too much at any one meal can lead to indigestion, particularly as you get older. Similarly, going without breakfast could lead to overloading later in the day; so if you really can't face something first thing, do try and have a bite to eat around eleven o'clock to prevent this from happening.

While I'm on the subject of breakfast I find I am quite frequently asked about the value of fruit juice at this meal. It is an excellent source of vitamin C, but if you take a look at the menu on page 52 you will see that needs for this nutrient are more than adequately met without the presence of orange juice. Excess vitamin C won't do you any harm, and if you like fruit juice then I can think of no pleasanter way of starting the day, but don't consider it an essential. There are other sources of vitamin C which can quite adequately cover your needs.

How important are hot meals?

Some people don't feel properly fed unless thay have had at least one hot meal a day, but their reasons for thinking this are totally without foundation. Cold meals can be just as nutritious, salads based on a high protein food, for instance, and so, even, can snacks, such as sandwiches and fruit (a point I shall be expanding on shortly). But it is true that the 'snackier' a meal becomes the more likely it is for my guidelines to be abused. Low nutrient, high energy foods, such as biscuits and buns creep in at the expense of other more wholesome items.

Lunch rolls and fruit are enough for lunch

Rolls and fruit are enough for lunch, so long as they abide by my guidelines on page 49. If you had two cheese and tomato rolls, an apple and a cup of coffee made with milk, the nutritional contribution to the diet would compare favourably with the cooked lunch which was suggested on page 52 (energy value $\simeq$ 700 Calories, protein value $\simeq$ 20.0 gm.) In fact, you could have a sandwich meal for lunch and dinner and still be very well nourished.

Another frequent accompaniment to the lunch-time roll is a pint of beer or a glass of wine. As far as nutrition is concerned the only significant contribution that they would each make is to provide calories of energy, and the same goes for soft drinks; however, they do add much in the way of pleasure, and if taken in moderate quantities they certainly enhance a diet without damaging its nutrient balance.

Milk is so often recommended as part of a well-balanced diet – and not surprisingly because it is one of the most nutritionally wholesome foods available – but can you manage without it? I know of so many people who find they literally cannot tolerate it. Well, first of all you can reassure yourself that it is not a necessity as the chart on page 52 will show you. The diet would still have met all requirements except energy even if the milk had been missing. And, secondly, cheese serves as a very good substitute for milk in terms of nutrients.

Who is not average?

So far I have been talking about the needs of two hypothetical figures, Mr and Mrs Average. Are yours the same? For most people in this country the answer is yes because the DHSS recommendations on page 172 have deliberately been set high in order to cover the needs of the majority of the population (the one exception to this is energy, a requirement which people can't afford to exceed, but I'll be telling you more about that in my chapter on slimming). However, there are a few who, mainly for reasons of work, do have different requirements. For instance, consider a weight-lifter. It is usual for such a person to weigh at least 30 kilos (5 stone) more than that which is recommended, but he would never be classed as overweight, just very muscly. In order to achieve such a figure his diet is of vital importance. He will think nothing of downing 6 litres (10 pints) of milk and eating 1¼ kg. (3 lbs. 3 oz.) of steak a day when training for a competition; in fact, plenty of nutrients, especially protein, are a must. At the other extreme there is the model who makes a living out of staying on the slimmer side of slim. Ask nearly any girl in this profession about desire for food and you will find that each is constantly fighting off hunger pangs. Their calorie intake, in order to keep so slim, is often below the recommendation, usually under 2000 a day and yet because of the job's strenuous nature it is important for these girls to have a good intake of nutrients – plenty of protein, vitamins and minerals.

Up until now I have concentrated upon nutritional value of

food and diet, but this is by no means the only determinant of what you eat as I well realize. Clearly if a dish or single item looks uninviting and has an unpleasant aroma you will not want it, so *palatability* is important. Similarly, any food which you cannot afford you won't be able to have, so *cost* is important, too.

Let me deal first of all with palatability.

Palatability

How would you like a meal of chocolate-covered locusts or witchedy grubs? The thought of them certainly doesn't whet my appetite, mainly, I suppose, because they just aren't customary. But for the Chinese, chocolate-covered locusts are a delicacy and for the Australian aborigines, witchedy grubs are part of the normal diet. And how often have you sat down to a meal of horsemeat? Never, probably, and the very thought of it no doubt makes your stomach turn. Eating of horsemeat in this country has been taboo for many hundreds of years.

Those are just three foods which would not meet with a very favourable reception in this country, but despite being unusual to us, they are basically very normal in another sense; for when they are digested they still provide the same nutrients about which I was talking earlier.

Energy and nutrient composition of some unusual foods

Food (88g/3½oz portion in each case)	Energy	Protein	Calcium	Iron	Vitamins
Horsemeat	moderate	good	poor	moderate	poor
Locusts	„	„	„	poor	negligible
Witchedy grub	poor	„	„	„	poor

NB: in each case good, moderate, poor or negligible refers to the quality of the source.

What about common foods? Can they ever be unpalatable?

If you open a can of peas you expect them to be green; peas are always green, of course. But not always, for when they have been canned they lose their green colour and become a dowdy grey. Not quite so palatable, think the manufacturers and back goes the green colour. If you were given a chance to get used to grey peas you might like them; who knows?

Palatability of food can also be affected within your own home. If a menu has not been well planned and you have given no thought to colour, texture or flavour, then the resultant dishes will be unpalatable; for instance, white fish with herbs and grapes, served with tomatoes, followed by blackcurrant cheesecake on a crunchy biscuit base is far more appealing than white fish with cheese sauce, served with cauliflower, followed by apple mousse and cream. There is no variation in colour, flavour or texture in the latter menu. Similarly, badly cooked dishes, however well thought out in theory, won't be very palatable and are therefore less likely to be consumed than ones that have been nicely cooked.

Clearly palatability can have quite an effect on what you eat; so, too, can cost.

Cost

'What the money won't buy the stomach can't have.' Today you are, no doubt, becoming more and more aware of this fact, as food prices rise at a very much faster rate than your salary. But does this automatically mean a diet of poorer nutritional quality? It most certainly need not; however, it is true that more of the expensive rather than the cheap foods tend to be nutritious so it does mean more careful choice of ingredients.

I am not going to talk about actual prices of food for two reasons:

1 because they are continually changing; and
2 because food prices can vary from one shop to another. But I am going to give you an idea of what foods are 'cheap buys' for energy and for the main nutrients (see table opposite).

In summary, the following foods which are cheap sources of several nutrients could be used as a basis for a shoe-string diet:

Flour, bread, oatmeal, offal meat, milk, cheese, beans, lentils, margarine, raw cabbage and soya flour.

It may be that you are not quite that badly off but are nevertheless having to think in terms of slightly cheaper varieties of

Cheap buys for energy and for the main nutrients

Constituents	Food
Energy	
Calories	Flour, oatmeal, bread, lard, margarine, butter, oil, sugar, rice, pasta
Nutrients	
Protein	*Vegetable Sources:* flour, oatmeal, bread, beans, lentils *Animal Sources:* pilchards, cheese, milk, offal meat, tripe, sausages, chicken, coley fish
Calcium	Milk, cheese, flour, bread, pilchards, tripe, soya flour
Iron	Curry, offal meat, beans, lentils, oatmeal, bread
Vitamin A	Carrots, liver, margarine, butter, cheese
B Group	
Vitamin B1	Flour, oatmeal, bread, yeast, yeast extract, cornflakes
Vitamin B2	Offal meat, milk, cheese
Nicotinic Acid	Any meat, milk, cheese
Vitamin C	Cabbage, green peppers, fruit juice
Vitamin D	Margarine, sardines

your usual foods and perhaps the nutritional quality worries you. Well, don't let it. As I said above price is not necessarily indicative of this factor; for instance, a rump steak is just as good for you (and far more tasty!) as a fillet steak, so stop worrying and start enjoying.

I mentioned earlier that individual food prices can vary a lot from one shop to another; if you have the time it would be well spent to 'shop around', but I realize that for many people time means money in which case it's probably better to just shop sensibly in your local supermarket. For instance:

1   Buy the shop's own brand of food, whenever possible. It will undoubtedly be cheaper than the well-known varieties, and the quality will be similar. Why not compare the two and see for yourself.

2   Whenever canned foods are on special offer buy them for your store cupboard. You never know when they might come in useful.

3   'Reduced' perishable foods are worth buying if you can make quick use of them.

4   Always make sure that you have a shopping list and that you keep to it! Supermarkets are rather fond of 'pushing' a particular product by placing it in a stratégic position. Don't be tempted!

Money can be further saved by economical use of fuel when cooking. Try cooking several vegetables in one pan by wrapping each in a piece of foil and inserting in the water. Cook more potatoes than you require and serve what you don't eat at one meal in a sautéed or mashed form at the next.

Plan your oven cooking carefully. Always try to cook more than one dish at a time, e.g. combine a stew and fruit crumble, even if you are not going to eat them all straight away. Dishes can always be cooled quickly, kept cool and then served either cold or hot (after a thorough re-heating).

Plates can be warmed by immersing them in hot water or by placing them, for a short while on top of the saucepan which is cooking the vegetables.

Plan your meals well in advance and buy only what you need. Food which is not used is money wasted and, of course, knowledge of correct storage, a topic which I shall be looking at in the next chapter, is vital.

There's no doubt that all this money-saving information will be particularly useful if you are elderly — a time when most people really have to count their pennies. But what exactly should you be buying; do you still require the same foods as a younger adult?

The nutritional needs of the elderly

The one big difference is the requirement for calories. As you become older your energy needs decrease, particularly so after retirement age. This is in part due to a general slowing down of your bodily processes and also due to reduced activity. By the age of seventy-five you need only about two-thirds of the calories you needed when you were twenty-five. But despite requiring less energy your needs for protein, vitamins and minerals won't have changed much, so it is important that your diet now makes particular use of very nutritious foods and avoids those high in calories and poor in quality. Here are some useful tips to help you achieve such an intake:

1   Have 300 ml. (½ pint) of milk each day (38 g./1½ oz. cheese is a possible alternative).
2   Have three meals each day and in every one include a portion of either meat, fish, cheese or egg. Try to have liver or kidney at least once a week, as a precaution against iron deficiency anaemia.
3   Have two or more daily servings of vegetables which should not have been stored for too long, chopped up too long before cooking, cooked for too long or in too much water, or kept hot for too long after cooking.
4   Have at least one piece of fresh fruit a day, and if you can't peel it, squeeze the juice (if it has juice to be squeezed!) into a glass and drink it or add it to whatever you may be cooking.
5   Bread and margarine can be included to satisfy the appetite but other high carbohydrate, high-fat foods such as cake and biscuits, should be kept to a minimum.
6   Always try to grill and bake rather than fry. Fried foods tend to provide too many calories, and they can also cause indigestion.
7   As you become older your sense of taste deteriorates and so you appreciate foods that have a distinctive flavour rather than a bland one. When shopping always keep this in mind; it will help to sustain a healthy interest in what you eat.
8   Keep yourself occupied. If you lose interest in life a vicious circle will develop, the more apathetic you become the less well you will eat and the worse you will feel and so on. Cooking and eating well can be a very fulfilling way of passing the time in retirement. Make the most of it, and if you don't know how to cook join a class. Many local authorities run them for people of your age group.
9   Try to get outside as much as possible. Not only will the change of environment and increased activity do you good but so also will the sunlight. Its action on your skin will supplement the vitamin D supply from your diet.
10   Make sure you have plenty of fluid. It helps prevent constipation and bladder infections, but if you think you might have

a problem during the night, remember to have your last glass well before retiring to bed.

11   Roughage from such items as wholemeal bread, vegetables and fruit help your bowels to work correctly, but if you have dentures you may need to chop these foods before eating. However, bran sprinkled on fruit juice or in a milk pudding should not cause any problems and will perform exactly the same function.

12   If you are feeling unwell and don't want solid food, nutritious drinks with a milk base can always be substituted. For instance:

Milk and Lemon Nog (two servings)

1 tablespoon of lemon juice
Artificial liquid sweetener
1 egg, beaten
1 pint milk
Grated nutmeg

Beat lemon juice, sweetener and egg well together. Add milk and whisk. Pour into glasses and cool. Serve sprinkled with nutmeg.

13   If you have difficulty getting out to shop, ask the help of your friends or relatives or have a chat with your local vicar. He should be able to arrange something.

As a stand-by for when you are stranded at home unexpectedly it is always a good idea to have a selection of foods in your store cupboard. The following form a good basic group — you probably have most of them already.

long-life milk	rice
packet soups	packet jellies
condensed soups	canned fruit
canned stewed meat	instant desserts
canned luncheon meat	custard powder
canned fish e.g. pilchards	blancmange
canned baked beans	canned milk pudding
instant mashed potato	cocoa powder
canned vegetables	dried fruit

canned tomatoes	sugar
cream crackers	tea
breakfast cereal	coffee
porridge oats	flour
semolina	salt

14   If you are overweight, should you slim? Yes, most definitely. It's never too late to lose weight, and if you do, your life will be improved both in quality and in length. There is no reason why you shouldn't follow one of the diets given in the appendix of this book. However, as a precaution do let your doctor know exactly what you are doing. He may get a little worried by an apparently unexplainable loss of weight!

15   Here is a list of organizations about which every elderly person ought to know:

Meals-on-Wheels

A welfare scheme provides a hot lunch in the home on either one or more days depending upon needs. Your doctor would be able to organize this for you if he felt it necessary.

Luncheon Clubs

These are run mainly by local authorities and not only do they provide a hot meal but also a chance to meet other people. Again, your doctor would be able to put you in touch with such a group.

Old People's Clubs

These are run by many organizations and help kindle a person's interest in many different hobbies by organizing talks and demonstrations and encouraging an exchange of ideas. For details of nearby clubs ask your local authority or vicar.

Remember feeding well, even in old age, promotes a *healthy* and *happy life*.

3 Pregnancy and childhood

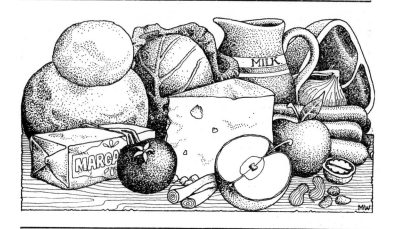

During the first nine months of life a baby is totally dependent upon its mother for nourishment, and if her food supply isn't sufficient she is the main one to suffer. A mother must not fall into the trap of over-compensating, either. This will not only leave her with an undesirable weight problem after birth, it could also bring with it unfortunate complications during the actual pregnancy. So striking the happy balance is what you must aim for and the advice below should help you achieve just that.

Eating during pregnancy

Consider the jobs you will be responsible for during this period:

1 maintenance of your own body;
2 growth and development of your baby.

During the first three months, when the emphasis is on the formation rather than the growth of your baby, your nutrient and energy needs will not be much different from those of a normal adult female. However, it is particularly important for you at this time to keep to the guidelines I laid down on page 49 for a well-balanced diet.

During the final six months, when your baby is increasing rapidly in size and extra maternal tissue is being formed, your nutrient needs, particularly for protein, calcium and vitamin D (the body-building nutrients required by your baby) and also your needs for calories of energy become greater. All these requirements can be easily furnished by including in your diet an extra half pint of milk and a slightly larger portion of meat or fish at supper, not as some like to believe by doubling up on everything that is eaten. In fact, this is probably the most important nutritional fact to remember. If you are pregnant, *don't* eat for two. After all, the baby you are catering for inside you is a good deal smaller than you and therefore doesn't need much.

Iron and multi-vitamin tablets are routinely handed out to most pregnant women. If you haven't been given any and wish to make absolutely certain of an adequate diet then your local clinic or chemist will undoubtedly help you. Incidentally, if you are pregnant and already have two or more children under school age you are entitled to free milk and vitamins from the State. Ask your doctor, midwife or health visitor for form FW8, if they haven't already advised you on this matter.

You may well find that you suffer from constipation during pregnancy. This can be due to a variety of reasons and is effectively counteracted by increasing the amount of roughage in your diet (roughage is found in foods such as fresh fruit, vegetables, wholemeal bread and bran) and by drinking plenty of fluids.

Morning sickness

In the early months feelings of nausea and actual vomiting quite often occur. These symptoms are all part of what is known as 'morning sickness'. This is a normal event in pregnancy and is often provoked by sickly smells, especially that of cooking fat. It can usually be relieved by just a cup of tea and a plain biscuit. Severe and/or persistent sickness should be discussed with your doctor, but no need for alarm, it does not indicate any kind of abnormality. He should be able to relieve the symptoms.

c

Bizarre cravings or pica

Thumbs down if you think you are entitled to a craving during pregnancy. True pica is really very rare amongst women living in Britain today. The cause is uncertain, but there can be no mistaking it since the items desired are truly bizarre – coal, for instance. In a recent survey a group of overweight mums were asked if they had experienced this symptom during pregnancy. The majority replied that they had, expecially for foods high in carbohydrate and fat such as chocolate and cake; a few did mention a desire for sharp-tasting foods like pickles which can sometimes occur. So much for the bizarre cravings of these ladies! Pica was just an excuse for most of them to indulge in their particular fancy and, predictably, it left them with a weight problem, which brings me on to the question:

How much weight should you gain?

Nowadays most doctors are very keen to check excessive weight gain, and if they don't, you should. To help you do just that here is a guide as to the kind of weight gain you might expect if you start off close to your ideal.

Weight gain guide during pregnancy

Time	Recommended gain
The first 20 weeks	3.5 kg. (8 lb.) – mostly in the latter 10 weeks
From the 21st week – the final week	9.0 kg. (20 lb.) – at a rate of 0.5 kg. (1 lb.) a week
Total gain	12.5 kg. (28 lb.)

A weight gain of 12.5 kg. (28 lb.) is generally considered to be the highest that is acceptable. Above that you will have laid down unnecessary fat. If you are on the smaller size or are naturally thin, then you will tend to gain less total weight. A lower limit of around 10 kg. (22 lb.) is recommended.

Can you slim when pregnant?

If you have more than 6½ kilos (2 stone) to lose (take a quick look at the ideal weight chart on page 96) there is absolutely no reason why you should not aim to keep your weight constant or, in the case of the very obese, to actually lose a small amount of weight during pregnancy. Do ensure that the diet you follow is of a high nutritional standard – the low carbohydrate one will probably suit you best; an example of this is shown in the Appendix C on page 174. During the last six months I would recommend that you include, in addition to the allowances stated, 300 ml. (½ pint) of milk or 38 g. (1½ oz.) of cheese daily.

If you have less than 12½ kg. (2 stone) to lose, but more than 3 kg. (½ stone), then you should aim to gain no more than 7 kg. (15 lb.) and again the low-carbohhydrate diet as explained above should suit you.

If you have only a few pounds to lose then my advice is aim to eat as sensibly as possible.

Incidentally, don't forget to tell your doctor you are slimming. He may become a bit worried if you don't gain weight as you should.

After the birth

This depends not only on adjusting your weight but also on altering the state of your muscles – something which is too often neglected. You should expect the former to return to normal within about a month, but it does vary from woman to woman. The latter is entirely dependent upon a religious adherence to regular toning exercises. In this instance it really does pay not to be lazy. Your doctor or health visitor will be able to advise you on the best routine to follow.

One final tip before I leave this subject: do keep trying on your pre-pregnancy clothes – you may have forgotten what shape you are aiming for!

Your diet

If you are breast feeding then you must take into consideration that your body is producing daily just under 900 ml. (1½ pints) of milk for your child, so it is obvious that you need a very nourishing diet, and the one you were following immediately before the birth would be very suitable. You must also ensure that you have plenty of fluid; its form doesn't really matter, so long as you don't go overboard on the highly calorific varieties. If you are bottle feeding, then I'm afraid no extras are allowed. It's back to normal eating, but with emphasis on a well-balanced diet, because those first few months can be quite a strain.

If you are breast feeding and see no chance of regaining your former weight then follow the slimming rules for the last six months of pregnancy (see page 67) but include extra fluid. If you are bottle feeding then you can follow a regular slimming diet (see Appendix C page 174).

Breast or bottle

It may be out of fashion, inconvenient or even uninviting but *breast is best* for your baby. It ensures an excellent diet for the first few months of life. That's not to say that bottle feeding does just the opposite, it doesn't and there are many babies alive and well today to prove the point. However, it is more difficult to regulate quantity of intake, and none of the natural resistance to infection, which the breast-fed baby obtains from its mum via her milk, will be passed on.

Normally, after a little adjusting, there should be about five feeds per day, starting the first at about six a.m. and the last at about ten p.m. Don't worry if your child wants to be fed more frequently. It is not abnormal. It is just hard luck on you!

If you are breast feeding you should let your baby suck for about two minutes on each breast at every feed during the first few days. Gradually extend this time until you reach about ten minutes on the fourth day. From then on you need make no further increases in the duration of each feed. Don't feel that your baby is going short of food in the first few days. It is during this period that you will secrete a very rich and nutritious fluid called colostrum, which also contains a good representation of your antibodies – the defence mechanisms of the body. After about the third day you will start secreting milk, whose average nutritional composition will change as time progresses and the needs of your child alter.

You may suspect that you are not producing enough milk. If this is the case do have a chat with someone at your clinic, who will be able to critically assess the situation and, if your child is being underfed, which is very unlikely, you will be advised to supplement each feed with some bottle milk.

If you are bottle feeding, you will be advised at your clinic on how it should be administered, on the importance of keeping all equipment very clean, and on how it should be prepared. Do double-check the latter point yourself and see that you are making up the feeds according to the manufacturer's instructions (note: to avoid mistakes put the water in the bottle first). The dangers of too much cannot be over-emphasized. After all you don't want to start your child off with a weight problem, do you?

Milk supplements

If your baby was born at full-term and you are breast feeding him or feeding him with cow's milk then it would be advisable to supplement his diet with vitamin D after about four weeks, usually in the form of half a teaspoon of cod-liver oil twice a day. Proprietary feeds already have enough of this nutrient added. Premature babies need it sooner. Additional vitamin C – usually taken in the form one teaspoon of fresh or concentrated orange juice before each feed – can be taken as a precautionary measure starting about one month after birth. In any event, your clinic will be able to advise you.

Free supplies of vitamins and milk are available to all children who have at least two brothers and sisters under school age. If you haven't automatically been given the supplements then you must obtain form FW9 from a Social Security office.

Solid foods

The normal recommendation is to wean on to solids between four and six months by substituting, initially in just one daily meal, a small amount of non-lumpy food for a bit of milk. Then gradually to increase this replacement in the middle three meals of the day only. Incidentally, he probably won't like solid food much at first so do give it to him before the milk when he is really hungry. The transition from milk to solids should be completed within about one month. Once weaning on to solids has taken place you should gradually be able to stop the very early (six a.m.) and late night (ten p.m.) milk feeds. When you do this however, do redistribute the milk your child would have had amongst the other three meals of the day.

One of the chief reasons for introducing solids is because the amount of iron in breast and cow's milk is very small and by about five to six months a baby's store from birth will have been pretty well exhausted.

Milk should still form a large part of your infant's menu and initially it will be shared with special non-lumpy food, such as cereal gruels and boiled vegetables, but gradually more and more family meals can be substituted. By about ten to twelve months he should be eating an adult range of food. Do, however, be careful not to add sugar or salt to his food. What seems right for you is probably excessive to him. He just doesn't want food that is highly flavoured.

There are no end of different varieties of tinned baby food available on the market for your growing baby. There is no doubt that nutritionally they are very adequate and, of course, they are very convenient, but you must pay for this commodity. However, a word of warning: some infant foods do tend to be a little sweet, so try and avoid these if you wish to prevent a particular liking for this kind of food in later years.

You'll no doubt find your infant enjoys a comforter (and keeps quiet too!), but do resist the temptation to plant a sugary-coated one in his mouth every time he cries. Not only will it encourage a special liking for sweet foods, but it will also initiate decay of newly formed teeth.

Growth

If he is of average weight at birth (around $3\frac{1}{2}$ kg. /$7\frac{1}{2}$ lb.) then you should aim at double that weight by five months and treble it by a year. If he is heavier than average at birth then he will probably gain at a slower rate and vice versa if he is a light baby.

By the age of five your child will be over half his full grown height which gives you some idea of his rate of growth before that time. Because of this his requirements for all nutrients and energy per unit of his body weight are very high. But on account of his much smaller size he apparently needs to eat less than you (at the age of one about fifty per cent rising up to about eighty per cent by the age of five, but of course, these needs can vary greatly from one child to another. He may be very active in which case he would require a good deal more and vice versa if he is very inactive). However, even though he is eating less in quantity, the quality of his diet in terms of body-building nutrients should be better than yours and plenty of high protein foods (particularly milk) should be included. You may even wish to supplement his diet with vitamins A and D by providing cod-liver oil, and vitamin C by providing unsweetened orange juice. This practice need only be continued until he is two; after that a good mixed diet will be sufficient to keep him healthy.

Feeding times

It's important to guide your child along the best route early in life so that eating correctly becomes second nature. A regular eating pattern should be your aim for him, although you will undoubtedly find that some days he eats spontaneously more than others. Try to feed him three times a day at breakfast, lunch and dinner and restrict, to an absolute minimum, eating in-between meals.

What if he throws a fit of temper and then dogmatically refuses to eat anything offered? Every mum has experienced it together with all the frustration and worry it brings. You should tackle such a situation by remaining outwardly calm, even if inside you are boiling over. Remove the food and don't re-offer or replace it when your child feels in a more congenial mood. There's no need to worry just because he has missed a meal. He can always make up for it at the next! In this particular instance it's much better to cure him of his tantrum than to see that he eats regularly.

You may find that your child sometimes goes 'off' certain foods. Again, there is no need to worry too much. The best plan of action is to just let the faddiness die a natural death. However, it may be wise to check that his diet is not suffering nutritionally. Take a look at the table on page 48 and note which nutrients the offending food or foods provide. Then find alternative sources for these nutrients and make a point of including these foods in his diet. For instance, a lack of green vegetables if continued over a reasonably long period of time may result in a shortage of vitamin C. To prevent this happening you could encourage your child to eat plenty of non-green vegetables (such as tomatoes), or fruit, or to drink fresh fruit juice each day.

If your child sometimes doesn't quite finish what he has been served then don't stand over him until he has. He may well have satisfied his hunger in which case forcing him to 'clean his plate' will only encourage bad habits later in life.

Five and after

I have drawn a line between the ages of four and five, not because the nutritional needs of children change drastically at this stage, although they do continue to gradually increase until adolescence, but because it's now that you no longer have complete control over what your child consumes. He's started full-time school, and it isn't always practical for him to return home for his midday meal. So just what does he eat when he is there?

Food at school

The important opportunity to teach healthy eating habits by means of the school lunch has not been overlooked by many countries and Britain is no exception. It is also a good way of ensuring that those children who might possibly be at risk obtain a very much improved diet than would otherwise be theirs.

The theoretical nutritional content is officially laid down in the Department of Science and Education's circular 3/66 and according to this all meals served in schools at midday should contain 29 g. protein (of which at least 18.5 g. must be animal protein) — just under half the day's requirements — and 32 g. of fat in all forms; they should have an average energy value of 880 Calories or about one-third of the day's requirements. Meals reaching these standards should automatically provide suitable amounts of vitamins and minerals.

That is the theory, but how does it work out in practice? The kind of meal that would meet these requirements is typified by the example given below:

An example of a school meal which meets the legal requirements

First course:
250 g. (10 oz.) portion of shepherd's pie
150 g. (6 oz.) carrots tossed in 12 g. ($\frac{1}{2}$ oz.) of margarine

Second course:
150 g. (6 oz.) portion of rice pudding
1 teaspoon of golden syrup

The trouble with school meals is twofold:

1 it is difficult to keep a regular check on their quality; and
2 it is not easy to keep an eye on how much is wasted by each child.

If you are worried that your offspring is not eating adequately at school for whatever reason, do discuss this with your parent/ teacher association. Tell-tale signs of under-nutrition could be consistent tiredness and apathy on return from school and persistent complaints about school food. However, if your child comes home and regularly demands plenty to eat, this is not necessarily a sign that he has been underfed but just that he has a very healthy appetite. Do resist the temptation – and his – to satisfy that desire with too many cakes or biscuits. Limit these, particularly if you see a certain podginess developing.

The other point you must be wary of is the tuck shop which is now becoming a part of the furniture in many schools but usually has limited hours of opening. It would be totally unrealistic not to allow your child any pocket money for buying food from such establishments, but it is a wise parent who exercises some restriction on what is handed out, and if you feel that too much is being spent on sweets then restrict it accordingly.

Once adolescence is reached, don't be misled into thinking he's greedy. He's not. He's just satisfying his very great needs for energy and nutrients. It will not only be the most physically active period in his life but also the time of a second growth spurt (the first one occurs very early in life). Because of these

Table showing average weights of children

Girls

Height (without shoes) cm	ft	in	Weight kg.	st.	lb.
110	3	8	90	2	13
113	3	9	103	3	5
122	4	1	114	3	10
127	4	3	128	4	2
133	4	5	139	4	7
137	4	7	152	4	13
143	4	9	169	5	7
148	4	11	189	6	2
155	5	2	211	6	12
158	5	3	233	7	8
159	5	3½	251	8	2
160	5	4	257	8	5
161	5	4½	264	8	8

Boys

Height (without shoes) cm	ft	in	Weight kg.	st.	lb.
110	3	8	95	3	1
117	3	11	106	3	6
123	4	1	114	3	10
128	4	3	130	4	3
135	4	6	145	4	10
138	4	7	156	5	1
143	4	9	169	5	7
148	4	11	185	6	0
153	5	1	205	6	9
160	5	4	231	7	7
165	5	6	257	8	5
168	5	7	279	9	1
170	5	8	295	9	8
173	5	9	304	9	12

NOTE: These are only average figures. If your child appears to have a large frame (i.e. broad shoulders and large feet) then allow up to an extra seven lb. and vice versa if he is lightly built. These weights include an allowance for indoor clothing (approximately 2 kg./4 lb. for both girls and boys).

two points and his comparative size, he will, in fact, need to eat more now than at any other time. However, it's vitally important for you to see that he satisfies his needs with well-balanced meals and not with too many snack foods — an eating pattern which would undoubtedly lead to the problem of excess weight, sooner or later.

Average weights

In the end the very best way of assessing whether or not your child is receiving an adequate diet is to keep a check on his size, and to help you do just that I have devised the table opposite, which is an adaptation of U S A figures, known as the Boston Standard. However, do always remember that these tables are only a guide; the shape you can actually see is undoubtedly your best indicator of nutritional health.

4 For better or for worse

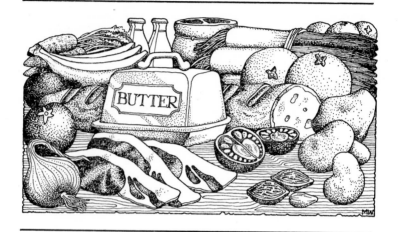

'Recently I have become aware of the "small print" on packaged and tinned food; for instance emulsifiers, flavourings and colour are often mentioned. What exactly are these things which are added to our meals whether we like it or not And are they really necessary?'

'My grandmother says that food isn't as tasty as it used to be when she was a girl. She says it's the fault of all those chemicals that are used nowadays. She thinks that in time we will all have so many chemicals inside us that they will do us harm.'

'As a working wife and mother I find I am using more frozen foods than I used to. How can I be sure that members of my family are still getting all the nutritious food I want them to have?'

People are worried about the manufactured food they eat, and the above three extracts from letters I have received recently bear this out.

Processing

Cast your mind over what you ate yesterday. I feel certain that you will have a hard time thinking of foods which haven't been altered or added to in some way by a manufacturer. After all just how many fresh foods do any of us eat these days? According to calculations about ninety-seven per cent of our calorie intake comes from those that have been processed outside the kitchen. Staggering, isn't it? But is it all necessary?

Undoubtedly, there are disadvantages, but these are more than offset by the advantages that are derived from factory processing, and chief amongst these plus points is the increased storage life which usually results. For if we all had to rely on fresh items as our sole source of sustenance we just wouldn't get enough to eat because there would not be sufficient to go round. Having enough to eat is not the only advantage of increased storage life; just think of the great variety of foods in your diet. This has only come about because of modern methods of preservation. Nowadays food can be transported to and from virtually any place on this earth; thus, in theory at least, it would be possible to eat anything that takes your fancy.

There is another important plus-point for factory processing, and that is that we rather like food which is so prepared. Not only does it taste good but it also doesn't take a long time to prepare. And, incidentally, this latter point is the basic ingredient of what are known as convenience foods or foods which have been largely prepared by the manufacturers. Not all processed items are as convenient as some others, but this factor seems to be rapidly developing amongst the manufactured food of today, as the housewife has less and less time or even inclination to spend in the kitchen.

So those are the advantages, but what about the disadvantages – the fact that nutritional value is affected and that additional chemicals are added to food? How do these, in practice, affect you?

I can best answer this by looking at factory processing in two parts: that which is performed by physical means, e.g. the application of heat, and that which is performed by chemical means, i.e. the use of additives. I shall start with the physical processes, but I shall only look at the ones that are in common use today. (Note: I exclude mechanical processing from this discussion because the only one which has any real nutritional significance – the refining of flour – is dealt with later on in Chapter 7 when I talk about white and brown bread.)

The physical processing of food

There are three main processes involved — heating, freezing, and dehydration — and it is these which are used, sometimes in combination, to make what you know as frozen, dried and canned food. From now on I shall discuss physical processing in terms of these three types of food.

There can be no doubt that the introduction of large-scale freezing, canning and drying has brought about a revolutionary change in your diet, and mainly because of their preservative action.

However, there is a price to be paid, and that is the loss of wanted chemicals. As the writer points out at the beginning of the chapter: 'How can I be sure that members of my family are still getting all the nutritious food I want them to have?' Physical processing *can* affect the value of food by destroying various nutrients, but so that you don't become too alarmed by all this let me just show you how your food is affected.

Cooking

Cooking is merely the preparation of food for eating by the application of heat, and I am mentioning it at this stage for one very good reason: I wish to show you that it, like processing in the factory, results in a nutrient loss, and it's worth your while to know how best you can counteract this state of affairs.

If you don't cook your food, much of what you normally eat would be totally unpalatable; it also safeguards against food poisoning because some unwanted microorganisms and enzymes are destroyed during the process. However, as I have said, it does adversely affect the nutritional value of anything that is so prepared, particularly if very high temperatures are employed with long cooking times, or if a great deal of water is used. The losses caused by the last factor can, to some extent, be redeemed by using the cooking water to make sauces or gravy.

Incidentally, microwave cooking, which does appear to be on the increase, although mostly in the commercial field, causes relatively little loss of nutrients and for your purposes is not worth worrying about.

Freezing

This can be carried out at home, although more usually it takes place in the factory. Its main aim is to prevent food from being spoiled by microorganisms, although it does also act as a time-saver in the home because all frozen food must be partially cooked or blanched, as in the case of vegetables, which means they are boiled in water or scalded in steam for a short time before being frozen. This heat treatment kills off all harmful bacteria and minimizes the enzyme activity of food before the freezing process, which is merely a convenient way of slowing down microbial growth and enzyme activity.

The main nutrient loss to frozen food occurs during the blanching process. However, this is not very great, and it would be fair to say that by the time you have finished cooking your own fresh foods they would be no better for you in terms of nutritional quality than if they had been frozen and then cooked by you; that is so long as you realize that the latter are partly cooked by the time you get hold of them and therefore you mustn't overcook them.

Drying

Drying is a very old method of preservation and works on the principle that removal of water from food will prevent microbial growth, enzyme activity, and most chemical changes, all of which would cause spoilage.

All vegetables, as with freezing, are blanched before being dried and thus a certain number of vitamins and minerals, which are soluble in water or are heat-sensitive, are lost due to this procedure.

The drying process itself can take place in a variety of different ways, with the aim being to dry the food as quickly as possible and yet do little damage to the nutritional quality. Normally about half of the vitamin C is lost and up to sixty-five per cent of vitamin B1 (or if sulphur dioxide has been added, which is reasonably common, there is complete loss of vitamin B1). With very prolonged drying methods (such as with dried fruit) a good deal of change occurs, but do remember that the foods which are subjected to this kind of treatment don't play a major nutritional role in your diet, and so it doesn't really matter.

Freeze-drying

This is a very modern method of food processing and, as its name implies, incorporates both the freezing and the drying techniques, by drying food which has already been frozen; a good example of this is freeze-dried coffee.

This process does cause losses of certain minerals and vitamins but not to the same extent as with the drying procedure, and, in fact, the freeze-dried product could be said to compare favourably with its equivalent fresh version.

Canning

Preservation of canned food also works on the principle of killing off all microorganisms and restricting enzyme activity by means of heat treatment, which may occur both before the food is placed in the container by blanching, and when once in the can.

As well as being treated with heat all air is removed from the container and thus a vacuum is created around the contents. Under this condition contamination from microorganisms is unable to occur.

Canning is a permanent form of preservation against microbial attack, unless the container is accidentally punctured or a seal breaks. Losses of vitamins, especially vitamin B1, folic acid (which is a member of the B group) and vitamin C, will occur, but precise values are impossible to give due to the number of different factors which can have an effect; these include air, light, acidity of food, size of can, and consistency of meat.

It would be fair to say that nutrient losses in factory food are, on the whole, very similar to those which occur in cooked 'fresh' food; that is, of course, so long as *you* remember not to overcook the factory food. I will now look at the effects of physical processing from the point of view of the individual nutrients.

The effects on nutrients

Protein.   Only if food is very severely heated will some of the protein within it be made less available. The same can also

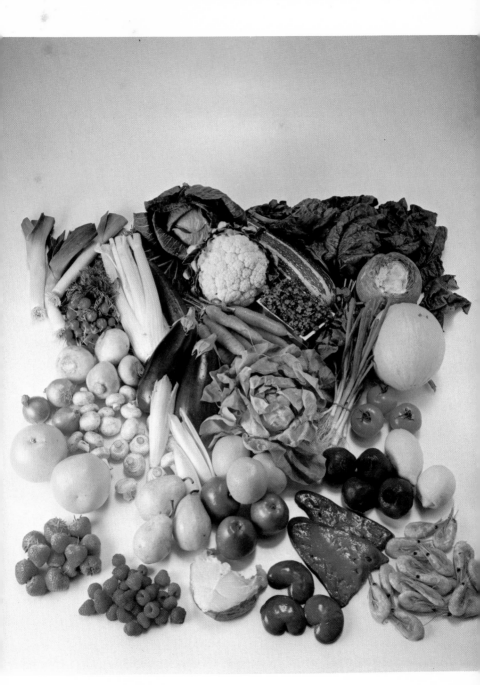

A 'slimming' selection

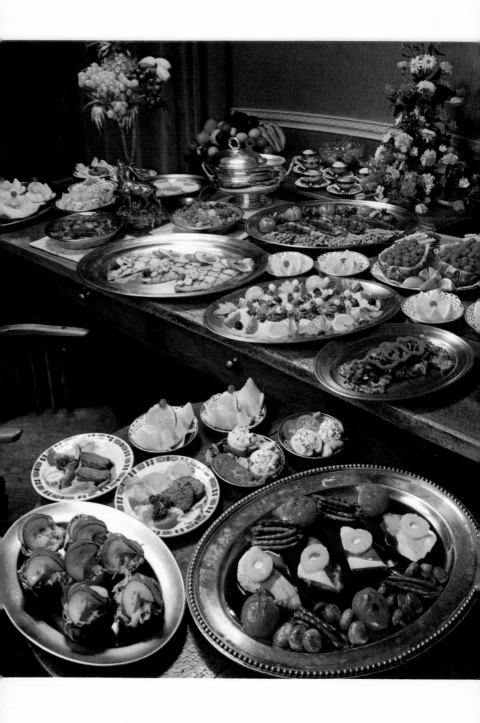

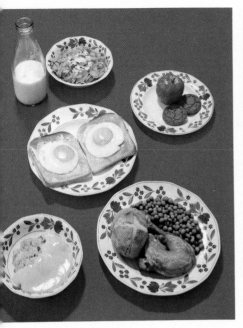

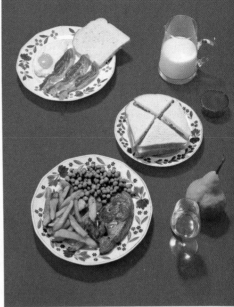

Daily diets to keep the average person
slim

Facing page:
Extravaganza in slimming style

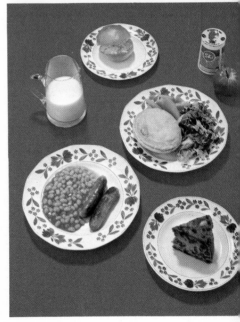

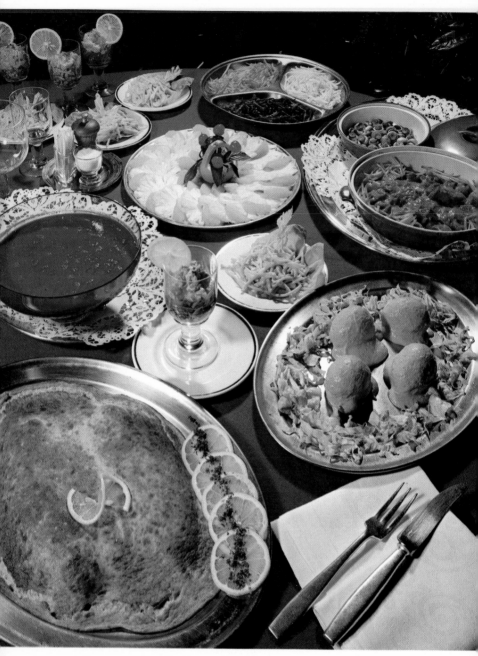

A mouth-watering menu for party-goers

happen during long periods of storage, even at room temperature. However, this loss is not really something you need worry about, because apart from anything else, you are unlikely to eat too much food that has been overcooked.

Minerals.   Minerals can leak out into the cooking water (which is one reason why it is a good idea to make use of the cooking water for things such as gravy), or they can leak into the water used for blanching food before factory processing.

Vitamin A.   There is some loss of this vitamin at high temperatures, in the presence of air or under prolonged storage conditions, if light and air are not excluded.

Vitamin B1.   This dissolves very easily in water and is thus easily lost during any cooking procedures which involve the immersion of food in water or the loss of water from food by heat treatment.
   Heat, if applied under alkaline conditions (for example, when sodium bicarbonate is added to the cooking water), causes great destruction of this vitamin. If applied under acidic conditions comparatively little is lost.
   If sulphur dioxide is used as a preservative then very little vitamin B1 will remain.

Vitamin B2.   It dissolves easily in water, but this is no real problem since foods containing good quantities of vitamin B1 are unlikely to be cooked in this way. It can also be lost in the presence of alkaline conditions, although it is not so affected as vitamin B1 by this factor, and it can easily be destroyed in the presence of light, so don't keep your milk bottles hanging around on your doorstep for too long.

Nicotinic Acid.   The only loss of this vitamin occurs when it dissolves in water, but this is not a very significant amount.

Vitamin C.   This is the nutrient most likely to be destroyed by processing. It dissolves in water, it is easily altered by air, by heat, by alkaline conditions, by the presence of certain metals, e.g. copper or iron, and finally by the release of an enzyme in fruit or vegetables, which occurs if they are cut. It is also lost during storage. But if the proper precautions are taken there should be no need to worry about an excess loss of this vitamin.

Vitamin D.   This is unaffected by usual methods of processing.

Precautions against nutrient loss

Certainly physical factors do affect the nutritional value of food, but so long as you take adequate precautions in your own home, you should have absolutely no need to worry. If you are eating a good mixed diet, you will be having more than enough nutrients anyway.

1. Try not to rely too heavily on reheated cooked foods.
2. Avoid over-cooking food.
3. Try to use cooking water or meat drippings as the ingredients for a sauce or a gravy.
4. Always prepare vegetables in the correct way: (a) don't keep them too long before cooking; (b) use the minimum amount of water; (c) cook fast and don't over-cook; (d) serve as soon as possible; (e) don't use sodium bicarbonate: it may improve colour, but it kills the vitamins B1 and C.
5. If you rely solely upon canned vegetables as your vitamin C source do include at least three oranges or three glasses of fresh orange juice in your weekly diet.

The chemical processing of food

The addition of chemicals or additives to food is not something that has recently taken place; although, admittedly, it has diversified its roles considerably over the last few decades. It has been going on for centuries; for instance, salt has been added to food as a form of preservation for thousands of years.

Additives do have their uses, certainly, and I shall be looking at these shortly, but as with physical processing there is a price to be paid. However, unlike the latter, where the price paid is one of losing wanted chemicals, the price paid for having additives is one of gaining unwanted chemicals.

Additives in your food

Have a look at nearly any packaged or canned food and you will find a list of ingredients written in small print on the outer surface of the container (incidentally, they are recorded in order of amount present, with the most abundant item heading the list). It can make surprising, some might even say horrifying, reading. For instance, I am told that the ingredients in a packet of margarine from which I have just been eating are as follows: edible oils, salt, whey, emulsifiers, colour (did you realize that margarine was coloured for you?), vitamin A, flavour (and flavoured too!), vitamin D.

Not all the above-mentioned substances are classed as food additives; only the ones which have deliberately been mixed with the basic ingredients (the edible oils and whey) to help make them into the form with which you are familiar.

Some substances have been added to food for so long now that they do not officially come under the title 'food additives' (e.g. salt), but those that do must undergo rigorous tests before they can be included on the 'permitted' list which means they can then be added to foods in controlled quantities by manu-facturers. (There is just one group of food additives, however, which at present does not need to be included on this list – the flavours – but it is hoped to shortly remedy this absence.)

All in all there are now about 3000 different additives deliber-ately placed in our food, and it has been estimated that each one of us eats on average about 1½ kg. (3 lb.) of them a year excluding salt and sugar (in comparison we each eat about 500 kg. or ½ ton of food per year). It's quite a sizeable intake of 'foreign chemicals' and not surprisingly the Government enforces the manufacturers of each additive to spend quite a large amount of time and money (approximately £¼ million) on safety testing.

Testing of additives

In brief, animals such as rats or guinea pigs are fed the sub-stance under investigation and are then examined for any harmful effects.

These feeding tests take place in three different stages. The first, which involves extremely large doses of the substance fed over a very short period of time (a week at the most), determines the quantity of substance that is needed to produce poisonous effects; if only a small amount is required then the manufacturers will not proceed with any further tests, and it would no longer be considered as a possible additive.

The second takes place over a longer period of time, approximately ninety days, and involves the testing of various different dose levels to establish an amount below which no adverse changes occur to the animal. It is from this dose that the quantity permitted in your food is calculated, usually about one-hundredth of the amount.

The third and final test is carried out over the long term (one to two years) on three different species to test for possible carcinogens and also for any untoward effects on the next generation.

In spite of these very rigorous investigations, no one can be certain that the additives on the permitted list in the quantities stated are one hundred per cent safe for our purposes for two main reasons. The first is that the tests, of necessity, must be carried out on animals rather than humans, and there is always the possibility that a substance which was harmless to the rat, for instance, might be harmful to you. The second is the problem of length of testing. Who knows, for instance, whether a substance, found to be non-carcinogenic after two years, might not initiate the formation of cancer cells after two years and a day? Of course, if it is not tested, no one will know. But even in the face of this uncertainty additives are allowed to join the permitted list. Why? Well, most of the decisions that we make in this life are arrived at by weighing up the options for a plan against those opposing it. If we don't allow additives we would be missing out on their many useful functions (which I shall discuss shortly), and it is felt that these outweigh the possible deleterious effects of their presence. Whenever a decision to allow an additive is made, the substance must not only pass the safety tests outlined above it must also be shown to play an essential role in the formation of a particular food or foods. It is in connection with this latter reason that many scientists are debating at present whether or not certain additives should be allowed. To find out more let's take a look at the different functions.

Roles of additives

These can be divided into three main groups:

The preservers.   Some prevent food spoilage by outside organisms (an example is sulphur dioxide) and some prevent spoilage from within (e.g. butylated hydroxyanisole, an antioxidant which is added to lard to delay it from turning rancid).

The improvers.   These are added by manufacturers in order to improve the nutritional quality of a particular product (e.g. vitamins A and D which are added to all margarines).

The enhancers.   The aim of all these is to enhance the quality of the final product. Some are considered to be technologically necessary (e.g. emulsifiers which are added to margarine to improve its texture), and some are felt to have only a cosmetic function (e.g. the flavourings and the colourings). It is this latter group of additives which causes some of the stir amongst scientists. Are they really necessary? For instance, do you need to have green peas in cans or can you make do with the grey variety, which would be the case if no green colouring was added? They'll taste just the same; it's just a question of getting used to the changed shade.

Nutritional quality

For practical purposes nutritional quality is not affected by additives. Sulphur dioxide, the preservative, does, however, adversely affect the vitamin B1 content of foods to which it is added but since their contribution of this nutrient to the total diet is negligible it's not worth your while worrying about a possible B1 shortage due to additives.

There is no evidence, at present, that the cumulative effects of additives could be a problem but this aspect is continually being monitored within laboratories funded by the Medical Research Council.

That's enough of all these nasty 'chemicals' which are added to our food — and note I have placed the word chemicals in inverted commas. Too many people, as does the dear grandmother who was mentioned at the start of this chapter, forget that all food is merely a collection of chemicals and that even we are of the same foundation.

Now we turn to some of the even nastier chemicals which occur naturally in the food you eat.

How safe is natural?

There are several foods available for your consumption today which, if they had to undergo the safety tests of present-day additives, would not be here tomorrow. Natural is not automatically nice. An obvious example of this is your dear old regular, the potato. It contains a highly poisonous substance, solanine, normally present only in minute quantities, but if potatoes are allowed to turn green then the amounts increase and could cause unwanted effects. As a safety precaution it's always wise to cut out any green parts which is where the poison accumulates.

There are also other naturally occurring poisons in food such as oxalic acid in rhubarb, or cyanide in the starchy root cassava. Even salt, that item you include in virtually every dish, has been shown to be harmful in doses that are much less than one hundred times the amount you eat. Certain vitamins are poisonous if you have too much of them (refer to Chapter 1) and, do you know, even too much water can do untold damage. Perhaps additives aren't so bad after all!

Processing of food has changed greatly since the early days, and there is no doubt that it will continue to change. Manufacturers are constantly striving for cheaper and more efficient methods that will retain nutritional value and not affect form (i.e. the structure, flavour and colour).

Storage

There is nothing more annoying than finding that a beautiful piece of steak in which you have invested has gone 'off' before you have had a chance to eat it. Annoying, yes, and, if you don't mind me saying, a little bad planning on your part. Food will only keep for a certain length of time (and I include the preserved varieties in this statement as well) and it's important that you, as cook, should know when that time is up.

Food loses its freshness because, quite obviously, changes

have taken place within it. These may be due to outside contamination such as from microorganisms, dirt or dust; from reactions between food constituents; from changes in enzymes; and, finally, from changes in the amount of moisture that is present; for instance, you are no doubt aware of how quickly bread will become dry and hard if it is not correctly stored and vice versa for biscuits.

Food will eventually deteriorate in quality however it is kept. This is an inevitable happening. But you can do a great deal to delay this process by storing under the correct conditions, for instance, the changes in fat which cause rancidity are greatly hastened by the presence of sunlight, thus it is a good idea to store all fatty food in a dark place and, of course, you should keep food in a clean environment to avoid contamination from dirt or dust. Correct storage is important, and it is worth your while to become acquainted with just a few facts on this subject.

Perishable foods

Foods which are classified as perishable are: all kinds of fresh meat, fish and cheese; milk; eggs; fats; bread and anything else made with flour; vegetables; and, finally, fruit.

Perishable foods can be stored in one of three ways: very short-term storage in a cool, well-ventilated, dry cupboard or larder; medium-term storage in a refrigerator; and longer-term storage in a deep freeze (and the ice-making compartment of your refrigerator).

It's quite likely that you have access to a larder and a refrigerator, so I shall take a look at both of these together and deal with them first of all.

I have devised a table which gives you an idea of how long you can expect to keep the different foods under these two conditions – that is, assuming they are reasonably fresh when you buy them.

Shorter-term storage life of perishable foods

Food	Refrigerator	Larder
Most meats	5 days	2 days
Mince, offal	2 days	1 day
Bacon	7 days	4 days
Fish	1 day	It won't keep
Eggs	3 weeks	2 weeks
Milk and cream	5 days	2 days
UHT milk	up to a year	6 weeks
which has been subjected to special high temperature preservation	(once opened treat as pasteurized milk)	
Cheese — hard varieties (e.g. Cheddar)	2 weeks	1 week
soft varieties (e.g. cottage cheese)	These will keep for a few days but ideally should be eaten as soon as possible.	
Butter	2–3 weeks (depending on brand)	1 week
Margarine	10 weeks	5 weeks
Lard	6 months	2 months

A few tips on how you can best prepare and keep foods in this way:

1. Do make sure that you don't overload either of the two places with items — air should be able to circulate freely.
2. It is usually best to lightly wrap food — this counteracts drying out and the mixing of smells.

These next few tips apply only to the refrigerator:

1. Don't leave the door open unecessarily, as this will raise the temperature inside.
2. Don't put food in when it is still hot as this will reduce its storage life.
3. Place the most perishable items, e.g. meat, near the bottom. This is the coolest part of your unit because cold air always falls.
4. Do keep your refrigerator clean.

There are some perishable foods for which storage methods are at slight variance with the above and are treated separately below.

1 *Oil.*   This can be kept in a cool dark place almost indefinitely. It should not be stored in a refrigerator.

2 *Bread.*   This should be kept in a clean, dry, ventilated bin and will stay fresh for about five days. Loaves with a crispy crust (such as the French or Vienna) should be eaten on the day of purchase. Clean your bin about once a week by wiping with a warm, soapy cloth and a splash of vinegar. Then dry thoroughly.

3 *Vegetables.*   Ideally they should be eaten on the day they are purchased, but if that is not possible they should be stored on a cool dark vegetable rack which allows the circulation of a good deal of air. Always see that vegetables are dry when they are stored. Potatoes do keep for somewhat longer than most other vegetables; however, their storage conditions should be identical.

4 *Fruit.*   The same applies to fruit as it does to vegetables. They are best eaten fresh, but if stored should be kept in a dark cool container. No fruit will last much longer than a week. Signs of spoilage will be all too apparent to the naked eye.

Now let me move on to storing perishable items over a longer term by freezing them, either in the ice-making compartment of your refrigerator or in a deep freeze, and I shall include in this discussion all commercially frozen foods since they can be treated in the same manner.

Storage in an ice-making compartment

There won't be much room in this compartment, and you will probably use it only as a storage place for commercially bought frozen foods, however, if you do decide to freeze perishable foods in this way, make sure they are properly prepared (I shall be running through this when I deal with preparation of perishable foods for your deep-freeze).

Length of storage life depends upon the type of refrigerator that you have.

The door of your ice-making compartment will have one star, two stars, or three stars printed upon it. This star-rating, as it is called, indicates what the temperature is inside and in consequence how long frozen food can be stored.

One star indicates safe storage for one week;
   temperature = 6°C (21°F)
Two stars indicate safe storage for one month;
   temperature = −12°C (10°F)
Three stars indicate safe storage for three months;
   temperature = −18°C (0°F)

When you come to cooking commercially frozen food do take note of the advice which is usually given about correct preparation once the food has been removed from the freezer.

Storage in a deep-freeze

A deep-freeze continues where the ice-making compartments leave off, i.e. food can be stored at temperatures of −18°C (0°F) and below.

As with storage in a larder or refrigerator, it is essential that you wrap every item. It is also important that you should label each food with the date that you placed it in your freezer.

Home-grown vegetables should be blanched — boiled in water for a short time (as are the commercially frozen varieties) — before being frozen. This minimizes enzyme activity which causes changes in the basic nature of food and kills off any potentially harmful bacteria.

The recommended storage life is limited, not because it would be a danger to health to eat food kept after this period (you remember, the cold prevents growth of harmful microorganisms), but because the flavour and quality of food gradually deteriorate with time; therefore, you might not be too taken by, say, some sausages which had been kept deep frozen for a couple of years.

There are many, many books available about storing frozen food and no doubt one came with your own deep freeze, but just to jog your memory I have drawn up an outline list of recommended storage times and I would suggest that you arrange as I have done below, the contents of your freezer into those that can be stored for one to two months, from three to four months, from five to six months, and from seven months and above. That way you will be less likely to keep food for longer than you should.

Storage life in a deep-freeze

one to two months	Any cooked meat Any kind of bacon Bread (crusty bread and rolls only about one week) Yeast pastries and pizza Meat casseroles, stews, curries, and pies
three to four months	Mince, offal, tripe and sausages – uncooked Giblets from poultry and game – uncooked Crab, lobster, and raw prawns Oily fish (e.g. trout, herring and salmon) – uncooked Cream Milk (should be frozen in a wax carton) Any cheese Uncooked pastry Soups, sauces and stocks Ice cream
five to six months	Lamb and pork – uncooked Duck, geese, turkey and game – uncooked White fish – uncooked Salted butter Baked cakes and pastries
seven months and above	Vegetables (twelve months) Fruit (twelve months) Beef – uncooked (twelve months) Chicken – uncooked (twelve months)

Eggs — removed from shell (nine
months)
Unsalted butter (nine months)

One final point on frozen foods: it would be wise not to refreeze thawed frozen food because thawing, particularly if it has been carried out slowly, causes a marked increase in the growth of microorganisms, and since freezing will not kill them, the next time you come to thaw the food it will probably end up with quite a large number of microbes within it.

Canned and dried food

Food which has been processed with preservation specifically in mind can be stored for a good deal longer than so-called perishable items. Unfortunately these do not last for ever. Even they are subjected to unwanted changes within themselves, both because of unhaltable chemical reactions and also because of changes brought about by the presence of micro-organisms, when they have been allowed entry through a crack or a split.

You can easily tell when spoilage has occurred. Changes in colour, texture, smell and flavour all give a good indication that this has happened. However, you would be well advised not to taste such food; it may well be poisonous.

Obviously this is important in relation to that list of cupboard foods given in the last chapter for old people; there were almost thirty of them and all very convenient to have on hand should anything, such as illness or bad weather, prevent shopping for a while. So let me show you just how long each should be kept in terms of four storage-life periods:

Up to one year.   Long-life milk, cream crackers, breakfast cereals, porridge oats, custard powder, blancmange, flour.

Up to two years.   Packet soups, condensed soup, instant desserts, canned fish, e.g. pilchards, semolina, rice, packet jellies, canned milk pudding, dried fruit, tea.

Up to three years.   Canned stewed meat, canned luncheon meat, instant mashed potato, canned tomatoes, canned vegetables.

Up to four years.   Canned baked beans, canned fruit, tinned cocoa powder, instant coffee.

Almost indefinitely.   Salt and sugar.

Keep things on separate shelves according to their storage lives. Whenever you buy new foods for your store cupboard always put them at the back of the respective shelf and bring the older contents forward. Do remember that once a tin of canned food is opened it should be treated as if it was fresh.

Hygiene

Correct storage certainly helps prevent the eating of unhealthy food, but other measures are also needed to be certain of such prevention, and they are usually associated with the way you handle food.

Did you know, for instance, that many of the foods you buy contain salmonella (a potentially poisonous organism)? For reasons such as this it is always wise to separate raw and cooked products and to always wash your hands when you change from handling raw food to handling cooked food. High temperatures kill off microorganisms so when in doubt always thoroughly heat food before eating.

Microorganisms grow and multiply much more quickly in warmth than in cold. Thus if you wish to keep cooked food for later consumption, cool it rapidly.

Utensils are usually cleaner than hands so always handle cooked food with the former rather than the latter. Do ensure to wash your utensils well after each use. They can support bacterial growth if they are not clean.

5 Overfed and overweight

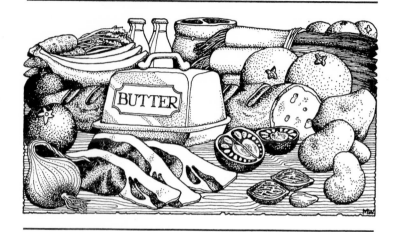

'Do you know it's making my life a misery?' said Mrs Bridges (vital statistics 42–34–48).

'Oh, come off it, surely not. You always look happy enough to me,' said Mrs Cope (vital statistics 34–24–34) in a somewhat bored fashion.

'Well, I'm not – oh, you just don't understand,' pleaded Mrs Bridges – in desperation.

To complete the story a dejected Mrs Bridges raided her full fridge and left not a morsel.

This little incident is so typical. Here is an overweight person, desperate for a cure, getting not an atom of understanding from a natural 'slimmy', and, in consequence, adding to her problem. Oh, yes, she knows she shouldn't have eaten all that food, but somehow she just couldn't control herself.

Losing weight successfully is so dependent upon you and your frame of mind. It is necessary to know a bit of theory but of far greater importance, in my opinion, is the strength of your will power, and it is with this thought very much in mind that I have written this chapter.

Are you overweight?

Quite frankly, most people know if they need to lose weight. Elaborate techniques are not required to determine whether you have a surplus. Certainly the first few pounds can creep on without you realizing what is happening but very soon their presence becomes all too apparent.

If you are keen on confirmatory tests then I could suggest no end of examples. I'm not going to, however, but I will give you three of my particular favourites.

The first of these is known as the pinch test – take some flesh at your waist between thumb and first finger, draw it away from the body and measure its width. You should come up with an answer of about an inch, this allows $\frac{1}{2}$ inch for fat and $\frac{1}{2}$ inch for skin thickness (incidentally men must allow themselves slightly less than one inch because ideally they should have just under $\frac{1}{2}$ inch of body fat directly beneath their waist skin). Crude? Yes! But it is a guide.

The second of these is known as the clothes test: do they still fit?

The third of these is known as the no-clothes test – strip off and stand in front of a full-length mirror (and if you are really feeling malicious jump up and down!) Do you really like what you see?

In fact, there is no real problem establishing whether or not you are overweight, but that is not all you want to know, I am sure.

Weight/height tables

Weight loss can be greatly aided by having a goal to aim for – a target weight. There is one slight hitch, however: how do you decide what it is?

The usual method is to obtain a copy of a weight/height chart and from it to read off what you should be. I have shown the most common of these, in a slightly adapted form, on the next page. It is the one compiled by the Metropolitan Life Insurance Company of America.

These tables can only ever be treated as a guide: in the end you are the very best judge of target. The reason for this is that

Desirable weight for height

Men

Height (without shoes) cm	ft. in.	Lower Limit kg	st. lb.	Upper Limit kg	st. lb.
155	5– 1	51	8– 0	64	10– 1
157	5– 2	52	8– 3	65	10– 4
160	5– 3	54	8– 6	67	10– 8
163	5– 4	55	8– 9	69	10–12
165	5– 5	56	8–12	71	11– 2
168	5– 6	58	9– 2	73	11– 7
170	5– 7	60	9– 6	75	11–12
173	5– 8	62	9–10	77	12– 2
175	5– 9	64	10– 0	79	12– 6
178	5–10	65	10– 4	81	12–11
180	5–11	67	10– 8	84	13– 2
183	6– 0	70	11– 0	86	13– 7
185	6– 1	72	11– 4	88	13–12
188	6– 2	74	11– 8	90	14– 3
191	6– 3	76	12– 0	93	14– 8

Women

Height (without shoes) cm	ft. in.	Lower Limit kg	st. lb.	Upper Limit kg	st. lb.
142	4– 8	42	6– 8	54	8– 7
145	4– 9	43	6–10	55	8–10
147	4–10	44	6–12	57	8–13
150	4–11	45	7– 1	58	9– 2
152	5– 0	46	7– 4	60	9– 5
155	5– 1	48	7– 7	61	9– 8
157	5– 2	49	7–10	63	9–12
160	5– 3	50	7–13	65	10– 2
163	5– 4	52	8– 2	66	10– 6
165	5– 5	54	8– 6	68	10–10
168	5– 6	55	8–10	70	11– 0
170	5– 7	57	9– 0	72	11– 4
173	5– 8	59	9– 4	74	11– 9
175	5– 9	61	9– 8	76	12– 0
178	5–10	63	9–12	79	12– 5

N.B.   These weights include an allowance for indoor clothing (Men = 3 kg./7 lb. and Women = 2 kg./4 lb.)

the weights shown in the above table are only the average weights of a very large group of individuals, so you can't be absolutely certain that they are the most healthy weights. Even if they are, you don't quite know where you should be within your range because body weight is not only influenced by body fat, which is what you are interested in, but also by all other 'bodily parts'; frame size of your skeleton can affect target weight a good deal. I might have taken account of this factor in the above chart as the Metropolitan Life Insurance Company did, but I haven't because there is literally no simple method for determining frame size, so it would have been of no practical value for you.

In spite of the shortcomings I would definitely recommend that you consult a chart before you start a slimming campaign. There is a wide range of weights suggested for each height, and it is very unlikely that yours should fall outside the limits set. All you need do is pick a weight within your desirable range and aim for it. Once there or even nearly there, think again. It may be that the weight you are aiming for is, in your opinion, correct; if it is not then don't feel you can't alter your target.

Skinfold calipers

These are sometimes used for estimating suitable body weight. They are usually considered to be a more accurate method of determination than weight/height tables because they only measure body fat as opposed to total body weight, thus they do away with the problem of frame size, but I have two reservations to make about their use:

1. They can only give reliable readings in the hands of an experienced operator;
2. They work on the assumption that a certain percentage of body fat is ideal, but the medical profession is not totally agreed on the value of this measurement, as I have already intimated above.

Middle-age spread

There is no acceptable excuse for a widening of girth with increasing age, even though it is the norm rather than the

D

exception. Ideally your weight throughout most of adulthood should stay the same (assuming it was correct to start with!), decreasing slightly in old age. However, let me be a little kind on those of you who have perhaps passed the point of healthy perfection and become somewhat used to a well-covered frame. The thought of returning to an early twenties figure may seem a little far-fetched. If it is then I can understand, but don't let it stop you from at least reaching the upper limit of your desirable weight range.

Establishing that you have a weight problem is only the first rung on the ladder to slimness. Next you need to know why you are overweight.

Compare yourself with a bank account:

Money in	→ Account	→ Money out
Calories from food in	→ You	→ Calories lost due to activity (e.g. walking, sitting and breathing)

Keeping at the correct weight is merely a question of balancing the intake of calories from the food you eat against the calories you lose through activity.

If your account is in the red:

Not enough money in	→ Red Account	→ Too much money out
Not enough calories from food in	→ You lose fat and become thinner	→ Too many 'activity' calories lost

And in the black:

Too much money in	→ Black Account	→ Too little out
Too many calories from food in	→ You gain fat and become larger	→ Too few 'activity' calories lost

There is however, one big difference between you and your account; being in the black is good, being overweight is not.

What's wrong with excessive fat? You can't find clothes to

fit, you feel ungainly, you lack confidence, you feel ugly, etc. The list is endless. You could no doubt fill in another twenty suggestions and still have more to come.

All the reasons I have given so far in reply to the question, 'What's wrong with excessive fat?', lean towards the cosmetic rather than the health angle. It's the way most people think when they are first asked the same question, for until there is a medical complaint directly attributable to your obesity, you won't immediately think of this condition as being a health hazard, but it very definitely is.

Information collected by a life insurance company suggested that if you are at least twenty per cent over your desirable weight (and that means being, for example, 68 kg./10 st. 11 lb. instead of 57 kg./9 st.), you are more likely to die before someone who is the same age as you and yet who is not overweight.

That's off-putting enough I am sure but just to emphasize the health risk, I am going to give you some further statistics, produced by that self-same insurance company for those they rate as being overweight.

You are nearly four times as likely to develop diabetes, two times as likely to develop cirrhosis of the liver (this applies only to men incidentally), appendicitis and gallstones, and about one and a half times as likely to develop cardiovascular and kidney trouble. In addition, you are more accident prone due to loss of agility, operations are more difficult because of the presence of mountains of fat, your posture is adversely affected, you are more prone to aches and pains, and as I said in Chapter 2 the likelihood of complications during pregnancy is increased.

It's an unsavoury message, I know, but unfortunately it's true. There is, however, light at the end of the tunnel; if you lose the excess weight there is evidence that you will be as good as new and all ready to lead a long and healthy life. So how about getting started?

Slimming – a successful approach

Motivation

Above all else, you must want to lose weight, you must really desire to become a slimmer version of your present shape. If someone else has done the desiring for you and rather pushed you into following a slimming diet, then it's quite likely that you won't succeed. (Take note, slimming pushers!) It's rather like giving up smoking. A half-hearted attempt would be a failure. You must really want to stop.

Very often it helps, before you begin a slimming campaign, to make a list of all the reasons why you want to become slim. For example:

Reasons for a slimmer me

1. I will be able to buy size twelve dresses.
2. I will have more self-confidence.
3. I could wear a bikini on holiday.
4. I won't feel so tired.
   etc., etc.

Keep this list close by you at all times and whenever you feel like straying from the straight and narrow, read, mark, learn and inwardly digest it! It's amazing how many people, during a campaign, lose sight of just why they are slimming and then gradually lapse back into overeating.

Another good tip is to place a picture of your overweight self on the inside of your fridge door – to act as a stark reminder whenever you feel tempted!

To know that other people can do it is very often a good motivator. There are many excellent success stories to be found in popular slimming magazines. Keep a few of these as reading material for when you feel down. If they can do it, so can you.

Keeping a diary

Just to bring the message home, before you start slimming, that perhaps you have not been eating like a bird, keep a record of all that you have to eat and drink over a three-day period and then, if you have access to such information, make a note of the calorie content.

A somewhat overweight friend of mine had done this, and she sheepishly showed me the results. Opposite is a copy of the 'worst' day, as she put it, but even this wasn't very different from her other days.

Diary of an overweight eater

Date: Wednesday June 22nd

Meal	Food	Approximate quantity	Calorie value (to the nearest 5)
Breakfast	Cornflakes	1 oz.	100
	Milk	¼ pint	90
	Sugar	½ oz.	55
	Bacon	2 slices streaky fried	170
	Egg	1, fried	130
	Tomatoes	1, fried	40
	Toast	2 slices	140
	Butter	1 oz.	225
	Marmalade	2 oz.	145
	Tea and milk	4 fl. oz. (milk)	75
	Sugar	½ oz.	55
	Total		1225
Mid-Morning	Milky coffee	¼ pint of milk	90
	Chocolate biscuits	2	140
	Total		230
Lunch	Roast Pork	4 oz.	515
	Roast potatoes	4 oz.	220
	Peas	3 oz.	40
	Sprouts	3 oz.	15
	Jam Sponge and Custard	5 oz. ¼ pint	565
	Coffee and Cream	½ fl. oz. (cream)	30
	Total		1385
Mid-Afternoon	Tea and Milk	2 fl. oz (milk)	35
	Sugar	¼ oz.	30
	Total		65
Dinner	Soup	6 fl. oz.	115
	Scampi	6 oz.	360
	Chips	4 oz.	200
	Celery	6 oz.	5
	Cheesecake	3 oz.	450
	Cheese	2 oz.	240
	Biscuits	3	90
	Butter	1 oz.	225
	Coffee and Cream	1 fl. oz.	60
	Total		1745
	GRAND TOTAL		4650

No more motivation was needed to start this girl slimming. In fact, she still keeps a copy of the above to remind herself what not to do!

Diary keeping whilst losing weight can be extremely helpful, too. If you haven't been losing weight very well then keep a record of all you eat and drink for a week, in much the same fashion as above – although I trust with not the same intake! It will help put you back on the losing track.

Which diet?

You have two major choices:
1 Calorie-controlled;
2 Carbohydrate-controlled.

Never mix the two.

To explain the difference, I'll return to basics. The only way you can lose weight is if the food you eat provides you with less calories than the amount your body expends. In other words your body has a negative account of ready calories, so it must call on its fat store (which is the storage depot for calories in your body) to make up the balance.

The method by which the low-calorie diet achieves a weight loss is explained in its title; quite simply it reduces the number of calories into the body by cutting food intake. This kind of diet usually involves just a general cut-down of the normal diet, so you can still include that bar of chocolate or pint of beer if you want, but it does mean a very strict adherence to quantities.

The low-carbohydrate diet again works on the principle of reducing calorie intake, but in a slightly more devious way. As you already know the three main energy (calorie)-giving nutrients in the food you eat are: fats, carbohydrates and, to a lesser extent, protein. Normally approximately half of your calorie intake would come from carbohydrate, and the foods which are a rich source of this nutrient don't tend to make a very big contribution to the overall nutritional value of what you eat. By cutting your intake of high carbohydrate foods, e.g. bread, biscuits and potatoes, you should automatically cut your intake of calories without affecting the nutritional value of your diet too much. One further point: high carbohydrate foods tend to be carriers of high-fat foods, e.g. bread and butter, therefore your intake of fat, another rich source of calories, should automatically be reduced by this method of dieting. That is the theory. In practice it has been known for a person to have a 300 ml. (½ pint) pot of cream daily and to let his intake of high protein foods get a little out of control, with the result being no weight loss. So although this diet has the advantage of greater flexibility, mistakes are more likely to occur.

The choice is yours, but to help you make a decision I have drawn up a simple table showing you the main differences between the two diet systems.

Major differences between each diet system

Calorie-controlled	*Carbohydrate-controlled*
1 Exact quantities of food must be kept but no food need be excluded.	1 High protein and fatty foods need not be restricted but there is virtual exclusion of high carbohydrate foods from the diet.
2 It is a very-disciplined regime.	2 It is a more flexible regime.
3 It is difficult to follow if you cannot plan your own meals.	3 Because of its flexibility meal planning is no real problem.
4 Sweet food can be included.	4 Sweet food is virtually excluded

Both work if they are correctly followed but the low-carbohydrate diet, because of its lack of discipline and liberal allowance of fats, is less good for someone with not much to lose – say less than two stone.

How many calories?

Mr and Mrs Average need 2700 and 2200 daily Calories respectively in order to keep their weight steady. (This requirement would be higher if you were a bigger body size or more active than the average and vice versa if you were smaller or less active.) To lose weight (i.e. body fat) you need to reduce the above-mentioned calorie intake, but not too much at first. This is for two reasons: 1) your body becomes accustomed to a lower calorie intake and uses what it receives more efficiently; 2) your body size will hopefully continue to shrink and thus you need gradually less and less calories. It is therefore better to commence on a reaonably generous diet, so that you can cut back, if necessary, as you approach target.

If you have a good deal of weight to lose don't immediately decide on a very low target. Be more realistic about things; aim, perhaps, just a couple of stone lower for a weight that is within your grasp; once there you can reassess the situation.

The slimmers guide to calorie intake

Weight to Lose

Sex	*More than 13 kg. (2 stone)*	*Between 13 & 6 kg. (2 & 1 stone)*	*Less than 6 kg. (1 stone)*
Male	1750 calories	1500 calories	1250 calories
Female	1500 calories	1250 calories	1000 calories

Slimming plans

I have devised two slimming plans, one based on the low-calorie system and one of the low-carbohydrate system. These are both to be found in Appendix C on pages 174–180.

The calorie value of the first diet can be adapted according to requirement. You don't need to worry about calories, if you are following the second diet but always remember, in the back of your mind, that foods rich in energy, such as margarine, cream and oil should be treated with caution.

If you are following a calorie-controlled diet you will undoubtedly become acquainted with more and more calorie values of foods (there is a brief calorie and carbohydrate guide in Appendix A). This can only be a good thing and there is no reason why you should not substitute more and more of your own food ideas in my diet plan – so long as you bear nutrition in mind – and, perhaps, eventually, devise your own diet by calorie counting. If you do, remember to keep accurate records of what you have eaten. It's all too easy to forget what has gone before!

Vital statistics and scales

Keep a check on your progress by recording your weight loss and vital statistics on a chart. Remember that weight includes all parts of your body and not just your fat, which is what you are really interested in.

Bodily water levels which are also measured on the scales can fluctuate by up to 1 or 1½ kg. (3 lb. or 4 lb.) each day and from day to day so keep to the following simple rules to prevent disappointment at weigh-in time: only weigh yourself once a week and at the same time of day each time.

Your very first week of slimming will probably result in a high weight decrease, due to an abnormally large water loss associated with the reduction in your carbohydrate intake. Your body's fluid levels will readjust themselves during the second week which will in consequence mean only a poor loss on the scales, I'm afraid.

Your behaviour

Psychologists have been studying how they can help overweight people to slim and amongst other things they have come up with a process entitled 'Behaviour Modification'.

Overweight people, they have found, tend to react differently to food than their slim counterparts. Thus by altering the behaviour of the overweight so that it is more in line with that of the slim, the problem of excess eating may be reduced.

I have drawn up a list of ideas which you may wish to try, but do remember to keep working at them; after all, your present behaviour did not appear overnight.

Ways to modify behaviour

1. Eat more slowly.
2. Only eat when sitting at a table which has been properly laid for a meal.
3. Only drink when you have no food in your mouth.
4. Don't eat when watching television.
5. Always serve yourself less food than you think you might require, leaving the rest in the pot.

6. Keep all food wrapped and/or in tins; thus giving you extra time to think whether you really need to eat.

Your aim should be to eat and enjoy food, *not* to eat and *eat* it.

Exercise

How many overweight professional sportsmen do you know? None probably. In fact, think of anyone who regularly takes plenty of exercise. Is he overweight? All evidence to date shows that he is unlikely to be affected by a weight problem.

Extra exercise increases the number of calories lost from the body, thus it can help you to slim, but only if you don't eat more in compensation. It is for this latter reason that many slimmers say to me, 'I don't take any extra exercise because it makes me eat too much.' Is their complaint justified? Possibly, if they suddenly decide to go for a long, energetic walk and then do not rise from a chair for a further ten weeks. They eat to compensate for the walk and then they continue to eat a good deal because they have very rapidly become used to eating more. But if they take regular exercise, they should find that far from encouraging them to eat in excess it will actually help them to stick to a slimming diet.

How often have you overeaten when feeling tensed, fed-up or bored? Probably too many times to recount. Exercise can remedy the situation for you. It has a marvellously calming influence on people, and it also occupies time, thus preventing boredom.

Which exercise is best? Firstly, remember that you are fairly unfit and therefore must not overdo things initially, and secondly, remember that it's far better to start with something to which you will keep and not stop before too long. I feel there is no better way to exercise yourself than with a regular brisk daily walk, lasting about twenty minutes to half an hour; it's not too strenuous and not too irksome.

Physical jerks

Lift your right leg up, slowly, hold 1–2–3, and down, then do the same with the left leg, 10 minutes in the morning and 10 minutes at night.

How much do these kind of exercises help? Again, they will burn up extra calories of energy, but they are probably more beneficial for toning slackened muscles. I would definitely encourage you to keep a regular routine while dieting. It could make all the difference once you are slim. If you don't know which exercises to do, the following association should be able to help:

The Keep Fit Association
70 Brompton Road
London SW2
Telephone 01–584 3271

Stretch marks, which occur very often as a result of pregnancy, can possibly be helped by toning exercises, but I'm afraid prevention is *very* much better than cure in this particular instance: don't become too overweight during pregnancy in the first place.

Artificial aids

Slimming pills

Under prescription from your doctor, slimming pills should only ever be treated as a short-term booster. If you have got stuck, they may get you moving again but no more. Pills and potions bought over the counter perform the same role but usually in a less effective way.

'Slimming' foods?

Notice I have put the word slimming in inverted commas. This is because these foods don't burn up your fat if you eat them; they provide calories and thus 'fattening power' like any other foods. But they are specially designed to help you stick to a lower calorie intake. They can be divided into three main kinds:

1. The ones which contain virtually no calories at all.
2. The ones which are merely a lower calorie variety of a normal foodstuff, e.g. low-fat spread, or starch-reduced bread.
3. The ones which are a whole meal substitute.

The first variety is always based on saccharin, a non-calorific sweetener. They include all artificial sweeteners and all low-calorie soft drinks. These items are a boon to the slimmer and may be included in unlimited quantities in any reducing diet. Please note, however, that a diabetic food, one which contains the sweetener *sorbitol* instead of sugar, is not lower in calories than the ordinary product.

The second variety can help so long as you don't eat the foodstuffs to excess and thus cancel out the calorie-saving effect they are meant to bring about.

The third variety, again, can help if you are the kind of person who really needs discipline. Each meal contains a set number of calories and there is no chance of cheating, or going wrong if you stick religiously to the contents. Unfortunately they tend to be expensive, they can become monotonous, and they don't really train you to eat sensibly.

There are points for and against, but please don't ever think that you can eat these meals in addition to an ordinary meal. It has been known to happen, and the dieter has just got fatter rather than thinner!

Maintaining your target

You've reached your goal and you want to stay there. it is possible, and you must believe that it is. An attitude ot failure will encourage failure. All too often I hear a lady say, 'I've lost it but I know I'll put it all back on again.' If that is the attitude she adopts then she will.

While slimming you undoubtedly had to change your eating and cooking habits. Don't now feel that you can go back to your naughty old ways. If you do, you know what will happen: you will return to your former weight. Don't allow yourself a week of treat eating after reaching target, with a promise to be good afterwards, because it's more than likely that you won't be. You are bound to have lapses, but whenever possible try to prevent them.

You should by now know quite a bit about food, so do plan your meals sensibly. And I really do mean plan. Make out and use a shopping list regularly and see that it doesn't contain too many high-fat, high-carbohydrate foods.

Cook sensibly; when frying (yes, it can be allowed!), grilling or roasting always use the minimum amount of fat. Most people use far too much of this high-calorie foodstuff. And, how about a less liberal dotting of butter on the vegetables? Again, it is not necessary.

You've probably amassed quite a few low-calorie recipe ideas. Keep on collecting them and, of course, put them to practical use; for instance, if you want a pudding, make one that is light and airy rather than one that is heavy and solid.

A final point for those of you who don't like wasting money – gaining weight means another set of clothes. Is that what you really want?

Slimming children

One of the saddest sights, in my opinion, is to see an overweight child being teased about his condition by his friends. You know what the odd careless remark can do to you: magnify that distress ten times and you will have an idea of how an overweight child feels in the same situation. Life can be almost intolerable for him, and if he's your child then you should help him as much as possible.

First decide on his target weight by consulting the chart on page 74, then decide on the diet. A child of nine or over can use either of the two diets in Appendix C but with the following alterations:

1. Allow an extra 300 ml. ($\frac{1}{2}$ pint) of milk or 38 g. (1$\frac{1}{2}$ oz.) of hard cheese each day.
2. School lunch may be taken instead of the diet dinner but the pudding should be substituted for a piece of whole fruit.

If he is below the age of nine then you don't need a set diet but do encourage an adherence to the rules for a balanced diet stated on page 49. Very often at this age tubbiness can be corrected by just a change to better eating habits. If you are encouraging your overweight child to slim do let your doctor know. He will probably be very enthusiastic and helpful.

Children don't find it easy to stick to a diet so do encourage them as much as possible. Award small incentive prizes, and make them keep a chart on which they can record their weight loss. If you succeed in slimming an overweight child then you can have done nothing better for him.

Anorexia nervosa

A recent survey of teenage girls between sixteen and eighteen years showed the prevalence of this very distressing disease to be as high as 1 in 150.

It occurs when individuals, particularly girls in their late teens and early twenties, take slimming to extremes and just continue losing weight well below their target. It is vitally important that any girl suffering from this disease should seek medical help, or, in the case of those refusing to take such action (as is often the case), help should be sought for them.

Outside help

The doctor and dietician can help you in an individual way, and the slimming club, whether it be commercial or under the National Health Service, in a group way. Many people find that the latter is an excellent adjunct to a slimming campaign. 'Without it,' they say. 'I just wouldn't have succeeded.' The very fact that you must report to someone each week and let a crowd of people know how you have progressed is enough to make the pounds roll off. Added to this is the cameraderie and understanding created by a group of people who are all fighting the same problem.

Slimming groups under the National Health Service are free of charge, and you can find out more by speaking to the dietetic department of your local hospital.

You must pay a weekly fee (which might not be such a bad idea when trying to lose weight) at a commercial slimming club (e.g. *Slimming Magazine*'s Weight Watchers', or Silhouette's, which all have popular magazines on sale advertising their whereabouts).

If you are trying to slim and find you can't on your own then I sincerely encourage you to give a club a try. It may well provide the help you need.

6 Coronaries, cancer and caries

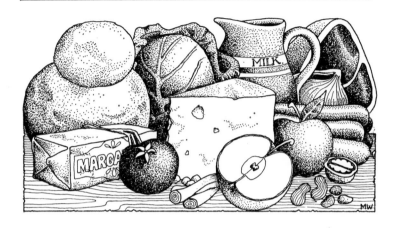

Not so long ago the most common deadly diseases were caused by microorganisms, but with the discovery of drugs such as penicillin and the success of various vaccines this is no longer the case. Now the chief killers are coronary heart disease and cancer. Unlike infectious diseases their cause is complex with a multiple of factors involved, whose relative contributions to the aetiology are still under dispute.

Not quite in the killer league but still very much a curse to health is tooth decay (due to the formation of dental caries) and gum disease. They have both reached almost epidemic proportions in the Western world and blame must rest largely with diet and standards of mouth hygiene.

It has all the makings of being a somewhat unsavoury chapter, doesn't it? Overall this is not the case: there is a wealth of positive information in the ensuing pages which can only help you to live a healthier and happier life.

There is nothing quite like a set of statistics for effectively bringing home a message. A record is kept of death causes by the Registrar General and in 1974 cardiovascular disease and cancer were very definitely the major killers amongst the middle-aged. Take a look at the table overleaf:

Causes of death amongst men and women in Great Britain between
the ages of 45–64 (1974) per 100000 of the population

Causes	Men	Women
Cardiovascular Disease*	563 (42% of total)	181 (24% of total)
Cancer	380 (28% of total)	300 (41% of total)
Others	400 (30% of total)	261 (35% of total)
Total Death Rate	1343	742

Above the age of sixty-four cardiovascular disease and cancer
remain the major killers.

The relationship between diet and coronary heart disease has
been much more extensively studied than that between diet
and cancer, and therefore I shall begin by discussing the former.

Coronary heart disease

Heart muscle, like all muscle, needs a regular supply of blood
in order to keep functioning. This blood is provided by the
coronary arteries.

Coronary heart disease occurs when these arteries become
blocked and in consequence seriously reduce blood flow to the
heart muscle. It can make itself known in one of three ways
depending on the degree of the blockage: angina pectoris, which
is the mildest form and is usually treated at home, heart attack
or myocardial infarction, which is treated in a hospital; and
sudden death.

Narrowing of the coronary artery is not a sudden affair. It
often starts at about the age of twenty in people from an industrial country; however, it takes some years before any
outward effects are felt.

Initially, a mass of fatty material, the main constituent of
which is cholesterol (a substance which is present in differing
amounts in everyone's blood), accumulates together in one or
more mounds just beneath the innermost membrane of a blood

*Cardiovascular disease includes a variety of different diseases of the
circulatory system, of which coronory heart disease, about which I shall be
talking in this chapter, is the main killer. It accounted for twenty-seven per
cent of the deaths amongst men and women in this particular group.

vessel, thus reducing its diameter. This is known as athero-sclerosis, and it can occur in any vessel but usually coronary arteries are affected sooner than most. It only produces disease when it blocks an artery supplying a vital organ which has virtually no other means of blood supply (e.g. coronary arteries, leading to coronary heart disease; and arteries of the brain, leading to a stroke).

Coronary heart disease usually occurs when a clot or thrombus (hence coronary thrombosis) forms above an atherosclerotic mound in the coronary artery – rather like the addition of a plug to an already partially blocked pipe – thus causing a very rapid reduction in the diameter of the blood vessel.

The ability of a person to withstand such a blockage depends to a large extent on the fitness of his heart muscles; in other words, if they are flabby they will be less able to cope with the sudden reduction in blood supply than if they were not. Fitness of the heart muscles is to a large degree reflected in the physical state of their owner – thus the reason for encouraging all inactive middle-aged people to take more exercise.

Risk factors

Coronary heart disease must be stopped; it is a major killer and is affecting people in ever younger age-groups. The aim of prevention must be to identify the risk factors involved and then to modify them accordingly.

To a large extent this has already been done but not all the factors identified can be changed. For instance, if coronary heart disease runs in the family then susceptibility is greater than normal; in fact, being born to the 'wrong' parents is probably the greatest single risk factor.

Men are more susceptible than women and they are most likely to be hit during middle-age. Also, if you have diabetes you are more susceptible. But even though these factors can't be altered, they can act as a warning to the 'owners' to pay particular attention to the factors which can.

The factors which can be altered mostly result from environmental influences which affect the affluent. This is known mainly because of epidemiological research (or in other words – study of factors and patterns associated with diseases). For instance, in Britain before 1900 coronary heart disease was virtually unknown as a cause of death, but since then, as we have become more and more wealthy the prevalence of this disease has risen dramatically. The only time this increase was not maintained was during the war years when things were a bit tighter all round.

If you studied the prevalence of coronary heart disease amongst a primitive community in Africa you would probably find no indication that it exists.

There has been other research too. For example, there have been many carefully controlled trials in which each suspected factor has been separately investigated. The end result was the conclusion that cigarette smoking, physical inactivity (as has been mentioned above), high blood pressure, raised blood fat concentrations, and obesity are all thought to be possible risk factors for coronary heart disease, but their relative contributions to the cause are at present still subject to much debate and discussion.

Since this book is entitled *Healthy Eating*, I shall confine my discussion only to those factors which can be largely affected by diet (raised blood fat concentrations and obesity), but don't think, therefore, that these are the key to the trouble because they are not. Cigarette smoking, physical inactivity and high blood pressure each play an important part and measures to counteract them should not be forgotten in any prevention programme.

The role of diet

Its part in the formation of coronary heart disease is by no means clear cut. Several different foods have been implicated; fat and to a lesser degree sugar are the two main ones.

The most recent medical opinion in Great Britain, in the guise of a report printed in the *Journal of the Royal College of Physicians of London* in 1976, certainy feels that the role of fat in the causation of coronary heart disease is the one to worry about. Some but not all would agree with this emphasis. The fat hypothesis does have the most positive evidence to support it, and for this reason it will be discussed first.

Before I do, let me just give you a brief explanation of all the different fats which are involved so that you won't be too lost by what I am about to tell you.

Fats in your food may be either solid or liquid (in which case they are known as oils), and they are mainly made up of substances known as triglycerides which in turn are made of up two different kinds of substances: fatty acids, which are what we are interested in here, and glycerol (or glycerine).

Fatty acids can be polyunsaturated (and fats containing large amounts of these acids are usually liquid at room temperature), monounsaturated or, saturated (and fats containing large amounts of these acids are usually solid at room temperature).

The fat theory

The connection between fat intake and coronary heart disease is thought to be as follows:
High saturated dietary fatty acid intake → raised blood cholesterol levels→atherosclerosis→coronary heart disease.

Firstly, there is evidence that when people with raised blood cholesterol levels lower their intake of saturated fatty acids and use only polyunsaturated fatty acid for cooking, their blood cholesterol levels fall and they stay low as long as the changed diet is followed.

Secondly, a stepwise positive relationship between raised blood cholesterol levels, atherosclerosis and finally coronary heart disease has been shown by several prospective studies, the most famous of which was carried out in Framingham, Massachusetts, a small town in the United States. It was a prospective study for coronary heart disease involving the selection of a group of so-called healthy middle-aged people, who were examined thoroughly and then closely monitored for signs of coronary development in the ensuing years.

No significant connection in these prospective studies has been found between the recorded dietary fat intake of individuals and coronary heart disease. However, it must be admitted that dietary fat intake is difficult to record accurately and that there are other factors which affect blood cholesterol levels.

A further kind of test has been carried out on a few small groups of individuals. It involves half a group following a diet low in saturated fatty acids and partially substituted with polyunsaturated fatty acids and the other half continuing with their usual high fat diet. In all cases the group following the modified diet recorded a lower incidence of coronary heart disease, but it must be remembered that the groups in each case were only small; for a study of this kind to be of real significance the numbers involved should be far higher.

The evidence is not absolute, but it has been strong enough to influence a medical committee (The Joint Working Party of the Royal College of Physicians of London and the British Cardiac Society) into recommending a reduction in dietary saturated fatty acids and cholesterol together with a partial substitution of polyunsaturated fatty acids as a measure of protection against coronary heart disease.

The sugar theory

Much less work has been carried out on the role of sugar in the causation of coronary heart disease.

The main argument here is that raised blood cholesterol is *not* the only abnormality associated with coronary heart disease; there are several others including raised blood triglycerides (these occur naturally in the blood and are used to carry fatty acids around the body), uric acid and glucose. Sugar does not affect blood cholesterol levels but it does affect the levels of the latter three substances which remain unaffected by dietary fat intake. However, it is still by no means certain what part, if any, these latter substances actually play in *causing* the disease.

So far most of the evidence to back the sugar consumption/coronary heart disease link has come from a number of studies which strongly correlate sugar intake with prevalence of the disease, though the same correlation could be said to apply to other factors; for instance, saturated dietary fat intake.

The Medical Research Council has carried out an official investigation into the sugar theory. They found that the victims of heart disease had slightly more sugar in their blood, but as they suggest the culprit in this instance could have been cigarette smoking rather than sugar because smokers, due to a loss of taste, prefer sweeter foods and thus eat more sugar than non-smokers.

I have explained in a very brief form some of the evidence

implicating both fat and sugar in the heart disease saga, but fingers have been pointed at other dietary items; for instance, salt, soft drinking water and lack of roughage. The evidence for these three and others is perhaps not so strong. However, it is of interest to note that so many different dietary items have come under scrutiny.

Coronary heart disease is not easy to understand; its development is indeed complex, hence the reason for much debate and discussion. But, of course, you can't wait until the factors are established beyond all doubt; you must continue eating while the search continues for newer and better evidence.

Your diet

I have said earlier that the most recent medical opinion in Britain is to reduce dietary intake of saturated fatty acids and partially substitute with polyunsaturated fatty acids, although it must be pointed out that the latter recommendation was not felt to be justified in another British report on the prevention of coronary heart disease (Diet and Coronary Heart Disease, HMSO, 1974). It does not feel that sugar plays an important part. However, it does feel that a reduction of sugar intake will help counteract obesity, which is associated with three of the risk factors: high blood pressure, physical inactivity and diabetes.

The extent to which you follow these recommendations is ultimately your choice and will undoubtedly be influenced by how much at risk you are but never lose sight of two facts: no one is one hundred per cent certain that these are correct; and there are other very important measures you can take, such as more exercise, to counteract heart disease.

Fats, fats and more fats!

You eat fat as a source of energy and nutrients. You also eat it because it makes your food taste good, but it's quite likely that you eat more than you need, and that you could, without too much difficulty, get used to consuming less. About forty per cent of your calories come from fat and this should be reduced to about thirty-five per cent or lower if you really are at risk.

Fatty acids

Dietary fats contain, as I have said, substances known as fatty acids; these are of three types — polyunsaturated, mono-unsaturated and saturated — depending upon their chemical make-up. For your purposes polyunsaturated fatty acids are thought by some to have a blood cholesterol lowering effect. However, they have been shown to increase a person's require-ment for vitamin E and there may even be a link between a high intake and cancer, so don't overdo them. Monounsaturated fatty acids don't seem to have any effect on blood cholesterol, and saturated fatty acids, if eaten over a long period of time and in large quantitites, appear to raise it.

Where do you find all these fatty acids?

Rich sources of polyunsaturated fatty acids (all of vegetable origin)	Rich sources of monounsaturated fatty acids (all of vegetable origin)	Rich sources of saturated fatty acids (mostly of animal origin)
tend to lower blood cholesterol levels	*do not affect blood-cholesterol levels*	*tend to raise blood-cholesterol levels*
corn oil sunflower seed oil margarines (which state specifically that they are a good source of this fat) cotton seed oil soya bean oil safflower seed oil	peanut oil peanut butter olives avocado pears	butter, margarines (hard), lard, dripping, suet, dairy ice cream cream cheeses (from whole milk) evaporated milk, milk fat, meat fat coconut chocolate, cocoa

Please note that not all margarines come under the heading 'Rich sources of polyunsaturated fatty acids'. In fact, very few varieties do. Only those which specifically state on the packet that they contain a good deal of this kind of fat are allowed, which rules out all the hard specimens and most of the soft.

If you are keen to use polyunsaturated fatty acids in your cooking, then oils are your best bet, but don't fall into the trap of buying ones which are somewhat anonymously called 'vegetable' because it's more than likely that they won't be what you are after. Always make sure that you buy ones made from an oil high in polyunsaturated fatty acids, as stated above.

Cholesterol

Blood cholesterol can be raised in two ways by dietary means: one, as we have seen, is by a high intake of saturated fatty acids, and the other is by cholesterol direct from your diet. This second supply is felt to have a much smaller effect upon blood cholesterol levels than the first source but nevertheless it should be considered if you are really at risk for developing a coronary.

Foods rich in cholesterol (all of animal origin) are:

Egg (from the egg yolk)	Tripe
Cream	Brains
Sweetbread	Prawns
Liver	Shrimps
Heart	Fish roes
Tongue	Stilton and Cheddar cheese

If you are still worrying about that egg you have for breakfast, my advice is don't, unless you have been specifically warned by your doctor that you are at risk, in which case about three a week should be your allowance.

Weight

If you are overweight all this talk about fat reduction is fine, but what happens if you are not? You still need a certain number of calories each day, and if you lower your fat intake you will need to obtain the 'lost' energy from other sources. The foods to increase are primarily the fruits and vegetables and secondly foods such as bread, potatoes, rice and pasta, fish, and poultry, and finally, lean meat. Don't ever feel that you should increase your intake of sugar and sugary foods to make up the calorie deficit; this can only be a recipe for ill health, mainly in the form of obesity.

Cancer

As I said before the evidence in favour of diet being a possible risk factor has not been nearly so well researched as it has been for coronary heart disease, but so far the preventive advice being offered is somewhat similar: reduce total fat intake. There is also a recommendation for increase of dietary fibre, particularly in connection with cancer of the bowel. It is thought that since this substance reduces the transit time of food constituents through the intestine there is less chance of cancer-causing compounds being formed. Most of the evidence for this is epidemiological; for instance, in Africa, where a good deal of dietary fibre is eaten, cancer of the bowel is rare, but in Britain where dietary fibre is definitely lacking, this disease is much more common. Not strong evidence, admittedly, but cancer and evidence aside, it would do none of us any harm to increase our intake of dietary fibre, if only to combat constipation. Doctors have also been successfully treating patients with diverticulitis, an unpleasant disease of the bowel, by prescribing a high-fibre diet. Clearly there is more to this 'waste' substance, which is mostly a very complex and unabsorbable carbohydrate, than first meets the eye, and it is as well for you to know in which foods it can be found.

Foods providing a good source of dietary fibre (roughage) are:

Wholemeal bread
Wholemeal flour
Crispbreads made from wholemeal flour
Bran
Course oatmeal
All Bran
Brown rice
All raw fruit except banana flesh
Cooked and canned fruit with skins, pips or seeds
Starchy roots such as potato and parsnips
Most green vegetables such as cabbage, beans and peas
Nuts

[Notice that all foods of animal origin are absent from this list]

Illness

If you are not feeling too well, then a diet excluding the above foods (except in puréed form, if it is possible) is very often prescribed, together with an avoidance of strong or spicy foods, all of which are likely to irritate your stomach.

It would include missing out an old favourite, the apple – the one that is meant to keep the doctor away if eaten each day, *but* which doesn't, nor is it thought to give such good protection against tooth decay. Its high sugar content works in opposition to the beneficial effects of its abrasive cleaning action.

Tooth decay

The foods you eat do have quite an effect on the health of your mouth – a point worth considering when you realize that no less than seventy-eight per cent of eight-year-olds in England and Wales have active dental decay, while seventy-five per cent over the age of seven have gum disease. For adults the figures are just as staggering: thirty-seven per cent over the age of sixteen in England and Wales have none of their own teeth left and of those with some remaining, ninety-nine per cent have gum disease.

Development of decay

To understand how the rot sets in, it's worth considering the structure of a tooth. (See diagram on page 122.)

The bone-like substance, dentine, is protected on the outside by a thin layer of very hard material known as enamel, and it in turn looks after a soft pulp chamber on the inside which has a blood and nerve supply.

The main predisposing factor for decay is an acidic concentration within the mouth. This condition is most commonly achieved by fermentation of carbohydrates, e.g. sugar with the help of mouth bacteria. Fermentation of certain carbohydrates also results in a layer of unwanted white material known as plaque, covering the teeth. This encourages the decay because it prevents the cleaning action of saliva from reaching the bacteria living within it.

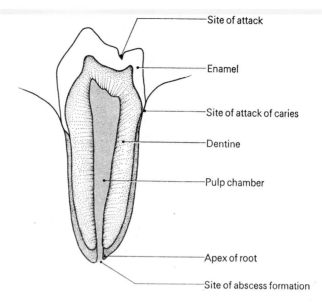

Site of attack

Enamel

Site of attack of caries

Dentine

Pulp chamber

Apex of root

Site of abscess formation

Plenty of fluorine, which is an element found within the dentine, has been shown to protect against decay, hence the reason for adding this substance to your water supply. However, a real excess can produce brown mottling of the teeth.

Once caries (decay of bone of teeth) are formed, the damage is irreversible. Certainly holes can be filled, an experience you have no doubt lived through during more than one visit to the dentist, but if the decay becomes too bad the whole tooth will have to be removed. Not much of a cure and, in this particular instance, it would certainly not be wrong to say that prevention is a *much* better alternative.

Gum disease

I mentioned earlier some pretty horrifying figures for the incidence of gum disease — a condition in which the flesh recedes away from the tooth and becomes red and inflamed at the margin of contact. Bacteria are the cause, and they are assisted in their job by the presence of an unwanted substance known as tartar.

Prevention

Prevention, as with tooth decay, is much better than cure, and not surprisingly the prevention is the same, so two birds can be killed with one stone.

It is so easy, but it does require a little work on your part. Firstly, steer clear of sticky sweets and soft, starchy foods between meals. They are particularly harmful since they lodge between the teeth and enourage decay.

Secondly, do visit your dentist as regularly as possible (say every six months). He can put a halt to any decay and rid your teeth of any plaque and tartar which may have accumulated.

Thirdly, if you are expecting a child you should realize that an inadequate diet could adversely affect the teeth of your developing offspring, so make sure you eat well when you are pregnant.

Finally, make regular use of your tooth-brush by means of a short sharp scrubbing action on each tooth, ideally for a good two minutes, after each meal.

It is probably the last of these preventive measures that is the most effective and yet so often forgotten. Without doubt early training encourages action later in life. If you have young children see that they carry out this very simple duty. It's in their interest.

The diet to cure all ills

I feel that a 'tying-together' is needed at the end of this chapter; after all, you can only eat one diet, not one for tooth decay, one for coronary heart disease, etc. and you may be just a little confused at this stage as to what that diet should be.

The rules for a balanced intake (on page 49) still apply, but knowing the many tempting diversions, let me emphasize three points:

1. Watch your fat intake (in other words, if you are used to more butter than bread, reverse the situation and remember the hidden fats in such foods as cream and chocolate);
2. Watch your sugar intake (and that includes sugary foods such as sweets and cakes);
3. Eat plenty of vegetables and fruit.

So simple and yet so healthy !

7 Alternative diets

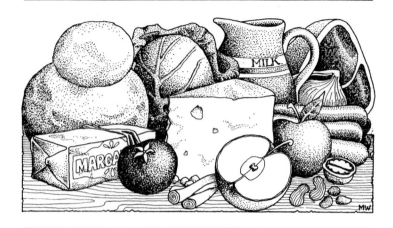

Thomas Adams, a Puritan preacher who lived in the seventeenth century, said: 'They have digged their graves with their teeth.' After the last two chapters you may well think that those words were prophetic. In fact, our present diet so worries some people — 'it is the cause of all ills', they say — that they have resorted to following rather different diets from the usual in an attempt to find a solution to the problem. Unfortunately, in their zeal to discover an alternative regime, they have often abused modern nutritional knowledge and encouraged people to follow a diet which is unnecessarily expensive and sometimes not in the best interests of health.

This chapter aims to take a look at the alternative diets of today and assess their real worth.

Health foods

The largest movement away from our present diet is amongst those who patronize health food shops and counters which have been in existence since the 1920s. Not all are vegetarians — people who won't eat any form of flesh, fish or fowl — but the health food regime is very much slanted in favour of a vegetable rather than an animal diet. It is felt that meat puts a heavier burden on the body's digestive and cleansing systems – something I shall be looking at later.

The health food addicts are very keen to get back to what nature has provided, with nothing added and nothing taken away. This 'natural' form of eating is best for both body and soul, they say.

The naturalness of health foods

The idea that foods straight from the field such as the whole wheat grain are natural is really pretty illogical. After all, who caused the wheat grain to be there in the first place? Man planted the seed. In fact, the cultivation of any plants can hardly be called a 'natural' process and likewise the produce cannot strictly be called natural.

However, the definition of natural is not an important issue in the health food way of eating. What you are really interested in is to know whether health foods are better for you than ordinary foods – which, incidentally, are far cheaper. The best way to discuss this is to look at just what is sold within a health food shop and see whether the claims made by the health food salesmen are justified.

Which foods are health foods?

Health foods can be divided into four main groups:

1. The 'natural' foods, or 'wholefoods' as some people in the health food trade prefer them to be called; foods which are as near to their natural state as possible, fresh and unprocessed;
2. Nutrient supplements, consisting of pills and foods rich in certain nutrients;
3. Herbal remedies, which are supposed to promote health;
4. Special foods which may not be 'wholefoods' but which claim to have special health-giving properties.
   Let me take a look at each of these groups in turn.

'Natural' or 'wholefoods'

I have already discussed the illogicality of the word 'natural' in the context of these foods. What their supporters are really trying to describe are foods which have been grown without the aid of artificial fertilizers, weed killers and insecticides and which are unprocessed.

It is true that these people may have a little something to chant about: adding extra chemicals to food, however well they have been tested, is not wholly desirable, but as we saw in Chapter 4 they are necessary if we are all to have enough to eat.

Doing without artifical fertilizers to grow crops would mean that yields would definitely drop below present levels of production. With no weed killers you would see more green than gold in a field of corn and without insecticides you would not only have less fruitful crops, but your diet would inadvertently include such delicacies as worms and maggots. The value of additives has been discussed in some detail in Chapter 4.

The wastage of food is high without the use of any of the above-mentioned manufacturing aids; it has been estimated that in the world as a whole about thirty per cent of food produced is lost by spoilage. It is vital that this wastage is combated if we are all to be fed.

Health food addicts, as well as being against the addition of chemicals, are against the taking away of parts of 'natural' foods. They claim that much of the goodness is lost by such an action. How correct are they in this assumption? To find out it is probably best to take a look at some of these 'wholefood' health foods and see just how nutritious they are.

Wholemeal bread.   Wholemeal bread is that which is made from wholemeal flour, NOT bread made from white flour which has been coloured brown, as is the case of so many loaves available today. You can easily pick it out by its very close, heavy texture, as compared with the light and open texture of bread made from extracted (usually white) flour. White bread is the very antithesis of all that health food addicts stand for: it is filled with chemicals and no longer in its 'whole' state. But is wholemeal brown bread that much better for you?

When the whole wheat grain is processed to make white flour, certain nutrients are partially lost and by law these must be added back to the white flour in the form of chalk, supplying calcium, 'powdered' iron, nicotinic acid and, finally, synthetic vitamin B1. Incidentally, there is no need to be worried about the word 'synthetic': synthetic nutrients are identical in action to their naturally occurring equivalent, despite all that health food addicts may say to the contrary.

The result of this addition procedure is to make white bread pretty well as wholesome as wholemeal brown.

Some even wonder whether all these additional nutrients are indeed necessary. A classic experiment was carried out by Professor McCance and Dr Widdowson, in which a large number of children, who would be the first individuals to show signs of a nutritional deficiency, were divided into three similar groups and fed virtually identical diets except for the type of bread consumed; one group had wholemeal, one, enriched white, and one, ordinary white. At the end of the experiment no signs of deficiency were shown by any of the children; they had all continued to grow in a very healthy way. The point this research really brought home was that if a person is eating a well-balanced diet it doesn't really matter what kind of bread is eaten. This finding is obviously of interest in connection with the type of bread to be eaten and, in the wider context, when it comes to assessing the true worth of nutrient supplements in a well-balanced diet.

So, for practical purposes, enriched white bread is nutritionally equal to wholemeal bread, but it does still lack dietary fibre, or roughage, the unabsorbable carbohydrate found in the outer husk of the grain. This is not classed as a nutrient, and its true value is very much under investigation at the moment. It is highly likely that we could all do with a bit more of this substance in our diet, but if you are totally wedded to your white loaf you will be pleased to hear that dietary fibre can be found in several other sources (see the list on page 120), so don't feel that wholemeal bread is a must.

Muesli. No self-respecting health food addict would go without his muesli, made from a mixture of whole cereal grains, with additions of dried fruits, nuts and raw sugar or honey – a totally wholesome meal. In actual fact, if its nutritional content is compared with that of a manufactured breakfast cereal and milk, it can be found to be of slightly poorer quality. Nevertheless, it is not an unacceptable way to start the day; it is just not necessarily the most nutritious, so don't be misled into thinking that it is.

Brown rice, wholegrain pasta.   All the grains, of which the above two are a part, are sold in their 'whole' state in a health food shop. As with the whole wheat grain which has already been discussed, the nutritional value of such items as rice and pasta is mostly to be found in the outer layer, which is removed on processing. Now we might have cause for worry, if for example, rice formed a large part of our diet as it does in many parts of the Far East, but the fact is that it doesn't.

An adult woman's daily requirement for vitamin B1, which is the first nutrient to make its absence known in a diet composed mainly of polished rice, can be obtained from the following foods: 150 g. (6 oz.) lean bacon or ox heart, 300 g. (12 oz.) liver, 137 g. (5¼ oz.) lean pork, 450 g. (18 oz.) enriched white bread, 112 g. (4½ oz.) peanuts, and indeed several other common foods are good sources. You can see that it is not hard to obtain a day's supply of vitamin B1 from a varied intake.

Wholegrains are a useful source of dietary fibre, a substance which has been discussed under the wholemeal bread section above; processed grains lose much of this substance during milling.

Pulses.   This is the name given to the family of dried vegetables which includes haricot beans, soya beans, chick peas, split peas, and lentils. They are all to be found in a health food shop, and it is true that they can be a cheap and good source of protein, but of course in a health food shop they are sold at a higher price than usual because of their 'natural' state.

Nuts.   Nuts, again, are a good source of protein (for instance, peanuts contain 8 g. per 25 g. (1 oz.) which is roughly one-seventh of an adult woman's daily requirement).

Dried fruit.   Health food addicts are incredibly fond of dried fruit, claiming them to be excellent suppliers of vitamins and minerals. Quite why they have achieved this fame is beyond me. Take a look at the table opposite:

Vitamin and mineral content of 25 g. (1 oz.) of dried prunes and
sultanas compared with the adult woman's daily requirement

Nutrients	Dried prunes	Sultanas	Daily requirement
Calcium (mg)	9	14.9	500
Iron (mg)	0.68	0·52	12
Vitamin A (retinol equivalent) (μg)	45	–	750
Vitamin B1 (mg)	0.03	0.1	0.9
Vitamin B2 (mg)	0.06	–	1.3
Nicotinic acid equivalent (mg)	0.4	–	15
Vitamin C (mg)	–	–	30
Vitamin D (μg)	–	–	2.5

(McCance & Widdowson Food Tables 1969 and DHSS 1969)

Two examples of dried fruit – rich in minerals and vitamins!!
Admittedly, they do contain moderate amounts of one or two
nutrients, but nothing particularly outstanding.

In their search to find nature the food addicts have strayed
somewhat far off the mark with the next group of items I shall
be looking at for, in order to produce many of these, very
complicated technology is required.

Nutrient supplements

There are literally hundreds and thousands of kinds available;
some are in a multi-vitamin form, some are just single vitamins
and some include minerals. The health food addicts claim that
these substances make the difference between health and ill-
health and therefore an adequate quantity must be included in a
'natural' diet. They are right up to a point, but what they fail to
realize is that a well-balanced diet will provide more than enough
of these nutrients, and that there is no benefit to be had from taking extra; in some cases, it can even lead to harm (remember the
vitamin A fanatic, described in Chapter 1). Very often they have
latched on to a rather minor vitamin and mineral and boosted its
ego out of all proportion.

E

Mineral and vitamin deficiencies.   It's true that in the early part
of this century, and before, mineral and vitamin deficiencies did
occur; diets were frequently poor. The table below gives you an
idea of what can happen if you go short.

The effects of a serious lack of the main minerals & vitamins

Nutrient	Effect
Minerals	
Calcium	Poor formation of your bones, leading to osteomalacia or bone which has become decalcified in adults, and stunted growth and rickets in children
Iron	Anaemia, which is also the result of many other causes
Vitamins	
Vitamin A	Night blindness, poor skin
Vitamin B1	Beriberi – a disease which involves weakness of the muscles, heart palpitations and degeneration of the nerves
Vitamin B2	Sores in the corner of the mouth
Nicotinic acid	Pellagra – a disease which leads to muscular weakness, mental and digestive disorders and dry, scaly skin.
Vitamin C	Scurvy
Vitamin D	The same as a lack of calcium

Nowadays it is virtually unknown for any of these deficiencies
to occur in this country. An incidence is only likely if the diet
has been seriously abused or, possibly, amongst rather vulner-
able groups whose nutritional needs are generally higher, such
as pregnant women and young children. But in the case of the
latter groups, protection is provided by the routine administration
of vitamin and mineral supplements and thus deficiency is
extrememly unlikely.

There is quite a fuzzy area between health and definite
deficiency which is characterized by the appearance of one of
the above diseases, and in such a state a person is definitely
below peak form. This could well be the case with some of the

elderly people in our community, but here the emphasis should be on encouraging them to take more interest in cooking and, in consequence, to eat in a better way, rather than on taking the short-cut route to adequacy by means of supplements.

A shortage – an intake below the recommended level – just will not occur for the average person eating a normal British diet, but can more do any extra good? As I have repeatedly emphasized, the answer is no, but how often is it that you hear of Mr Celebrity gulping down his ten multi-vitamin tablets a day and feeling fitter than fit on his regime?

Let me give you an example of how an excess of these supplements is supposed to work. The main B vitamins are used to release calories of energy from food. Thus, say the health food addicts, the more B vitamins you ingest, the more energy you will have. But it's rather like putting the cart before the horse, because your body will only release energy from food in response to the activity you have been taking. Eating more B vitamins, in the form of brewers' yeast tablets for instance, doesn't mean that you will suddenly start releasing more energy, nor for that matter will it help you to get slim by releasing energy stored in your fatty tissue. Your body will use what it requires and dispose of the rest. In much the same way an excess of vitamin A will not make your skin any healthier despite what the health food addicts claim.

Some of the minor nutrients, as I have said above, have become great favourites – iodine, for instance, an essential part of hormones produced by the thyroid gland, which regulates metabolic rate (the rate at which you burn up the calories of energy). It is implied that the more iodine you eat, the faster will be your metabolic rate and thus an excess will help if you are trying to lose weight. Of course, this is nonsense: as with the B vitamins, enough is as good as a feast.

Then there is that wonder of today: vitamin E. Its exact role has yet to be determined, and it's probably because of this lack of knowledge that health food addicts have seized upon the opportunity to decide their own ideas for its function.

In female rats a lack of it has been shown to cause resorption of the foetus about three-quarters of the way through pregnancy, and in male rats a shortage causes sterility. However, an administration of vitamin E to women who have had repeated miscarriages or to men who are sterile has been shown to have no effect. This is just one example of research that has been carried out on its possible function. I have explained it in a little detail because I wish to point out how futile is the claim that vitamin E has virility-giving powers. It has no doubt arisen because of the above research which, even if it did work with humans, has absolutely nothing to do with increasing your desire for sexual intercourse, a function which is implied in the claim.

Wheatgerm is the embryo from which a wheat plant develops and is a particularly rich source of vitamin E. It is available in its natural form in capsules, and in tablets, which gives you some idea of how much health food addicts revere this nutrient. An excess of vitamin E has not yet been shown to be harmful, but since it is fat-soluble like vitamins A and D and therefore, cannot be expelled by the body once absorbed, there is always the possibility that an accumulation may cause harm.

Herbal remedies

There is an abundance of herbal remedies, usually in bottled form, in any health food shop you care to visit. Herbalism is a centuries-old method of relieving sickness and could be said to have a very slight scientific backing. There are many, many different chemicals present in herbs and indeed in all plants, and it is just possible that some may relieve certain ills. But science has advanced greatly since the heyday of herbalism and now most of these chemicals have been isolated and improved upon. I have no doubt that a much more effective remedy can be found in a chemist's shop rather than in a health food shop.

Special foods

The final group I have called special foods. This is because they apparently meet the demands for certain food needs but aren't necessarily 'wholefoods'. They obviously deserve closer investigation.

Bran.   This is the outer husk of the wheat grain and is a very rich source of dietary fibre. Certainly there is no harm in sprinkling this substance on your daily bowl of cereal; it may even be doing you a lot of good.

Fats rich in polyunsaturated fatty acids. I have discussed how these are thought to be connected with coronary heart disease in Chapter 6 and listed possible sources, most of which can be obtained in normal shops.

Garlic. It has been linked with lowering blood cholesterol but this is not considered to be a serious possibility amongst scientists, and I would think that the only point you should seriously consider about this substance is the number of friends you might lose by eating too much!

Sea salt. 'Rich in minerals and trace elements, particularly iodine.' Do by all means have this substance, but don't think you need it for nutritional reasons, unless you are short of iodine, which is unlikely.

Kelp. 'Another sea-food rich in vitamins and mineral salts, particularly iodine.' Again, it's not nutritionally necessary but do have it, if you so desire.

Yoghurt. It must be 'live' and have had nothing added to it or in the words of the health food addict, in its truly 'natural' state. In fact, it is anything but natural since it has undergone quite a complicated procedure to arrive in its present state. However, it is a very nutritious food since it is basically milk, but its real value to the health food addicts lies not with its nutritional value (although that is reasonably important to them) but with the live bacteria it contains. These are supposed to replace those already found in your stomach and to aid digestion. This, I'm afraid, is rubbish. It is a fact that your stomach knows best in this particular instance and the yoghurt bacteria would be lucky to survive more than a few hours down there.

High protein drinks. These are not necessary for the ordinary individual but could be useful for someone wishing to build up his body, such as a weightlifter; however, there are more conventional dietary means of doing this.

Honey and other items. The bee and its produce has achieved a position of unique fame amongst health food addicts; the number of different varieties of honey in health food shops gives you an idea of its popularity. Indeed it is a very pleasant food to spread on bread, but has it any other attributes as implied by its supporters?

Most certainly, honey can have no claim to nutritional fame. Take a look at the table below.

Energy and nutrient composition of 1 tablespoon (25 g./1 oz.) of honey compared with a day's requirement for an adult female

Constituents	Honey	Requirement
Energy (Calories)	82	2200
Nutrients		
Protein	0.1	55
Vitamin B1 (mg.)	–	0.9
Vitamin B2 (mg.)	0.01	1.3
Nicotinic acid equivalent (mg.)	0.06	15
Vitamin C (mg.)	–	30
Vitamin A (retinol equivalent) (μg.)	–	750
Vitamin D (μg.)	–	2.5
Calcium (mg.)	1.5	500
Iron (mg.)	0.11	12

(McCance and Widdowson food tables 1969 and DHSS 1969)

About the only sizeable contribution it makes to the diet is in the number of calories it provides, and since there is very little nutrient contribution these calories could be considered totally unwholesome.

Certainly the wonder of honey does not lie in its nutritional content, but perhaps it can supply a health-giving drug. As yet nothing has been discovered and even if it was it is doubtful whether its effects would more than outweigh the nutritional imbalance caused by eating too much of this food.

Honey is very pleasant to taste so by all means have it in small quantities, but don't overdo it, particularly if you have a weight problem.

Equally as non-nutritious are pollen and royal jelly, which is 'the very rich food fed only to those who have been chosen to be Queen bee'!

Sugar. The final word must be given to sugar. Please don't be fooled into thinking that the unrefined variety is all right and that the refined is not. For practical nutritional purposes they are the same and neither is really necessary in a healthy well-balanced diet.

Vegetarianism

Most vegetarians buy in health food shops, mainly because these stores cater particularly for a vegetable-based diet.

Some people are vegetarians for religious and moral reasons: they don't like the thought of killing other animals for their own sustenance; some do this because they simply don't like flesh, fish or fowl; some do it for misguided health reasons, thinking meat releases toxins into the blood during digestion, which is not true; and finally some do it for a combination of the above factors.

There is usually no danger of a vegetarian going short of nutrients because he can include such items as milk, eggs and cheese — the very nutritious produce of animals. He can also make use of the vegetable meat substitute: textured vegetable protein. This is very nutritious, and we shall undoubtedly be seeing more of it in the future.

Veganism

This is a rather extreme form of vegetarianism and prohibits the intake of any food of animal origin which, of course, includes all dairy items such as milk and cheese. There is a possibility of vitamin B12 shortage with this diet, and a supplement of this nutrient is recommended. In order to obtain enough of all amino acids (the building-blocks of protein) it is wise to include proteins from a variety of sources, for instance, from grains, vegetables, nuts and fruit (see page 32).

Macrobiotic diet

It is a regime of relatively recent origin in the West, dating from the early part of this century under the 'divine' guidance of the great high priest of this way of life — George Ohsawa.

Macrobiotics is the Western term used to describe a centuries-old Far Eastern philosophy which adopted a system of restoration to health through diet.

All disease is apparently caused by an imbalance in the body of yin and yang, two forces which act in opposition to each other but are in fact complimentary rather like man and woman. All food is designated as either yin or yang; for instance, vegetables are yin and animal meat is yang, and the aim is to balance the two. Great emphasis is placed on whole grain cereals and in practice little else is eaten.

This diet totally ignores any of the significant nutritional findings of this century, and a report in the *Journal of the American Medical Association* describes it as a 'dangerous dietary philosophy'. Deficiency diseases caused by lack of vitamin C, vitamin B12, iron and calcium have been recorded as an outcome of this regime, and so even has death.

Not the most healthy of alternative diets, is it? Perhaps, after all, it is better to keep to the more conventional forms of intake. But as population increases at a faster rate than food supply, is there a possibility that we shall be forced to look for alternative forms of sustenance? This question is the subject of the next and final chapter.

8 Food for all

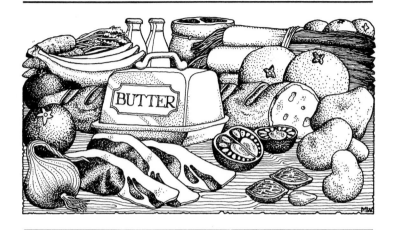

The idea that Britain might live through a famine is probably about as remote to you, at this moment in time, as the thought of taking up residence on the moon. This, I suppose, is understandable; you have probably never known a time of shortage and consequently you have been lulled into a sense of complete security; you expect the next meal to be on the table. But if the present population increase continues without effective intervention on our part and we make no attempt to change our present diet which is really rather extravagant in terms of natural resources to produce, then we might well encounter problems. But this needn't be the case; the opportunity to secure three meals a day for future generations is available, but we must take the necessary action now and not tomorrow.

The malthusian prediction

It was in the summer of 1798 that a young curate living in the country published his first work. He was Thomas Robert Malthus and in his publication, *An Essay on The Principle of Population*, he made the prediction that man's increase in numbers would soon outstrip his ability to keep pace with adequate food supplies. He was not, in fact, correct that it would *soon* outstrip supplies because, as yet, there has been no world famine, but it is not beyond the realms of possibility one day, as I have said above, if our population keeps expanding at its present rate.

The population explosion

Between the years 0 and 1500 AD population doubled every 700 years. This rate of increase then started to rise. A further doubling of the population was achieved after only 300 years and by the mid-1800s the total population was estimated to have reached about 1000 million. By the mid-1920s, less than a century later, it had doubled, and in 1963 it had reached 3000 million.

The United Nations have predicted, by taking into account rates of birth and maternal and infant mortality, that the world's population will reach somewhere between 6000 and 7000 million by 2000 AD.

The reason for this rapid increase in population has nothing to do with an increase in birth rate, which more recently in the industrialized world has been on the decline, but it has a great deal to do with the fall in death rate, and the reasons for this are somewhat complex.

In Britain Sir Hugh Myddelton, who in 1613 caused London to have a vastly improved water supply, did much to set the ball rolling. It was this emphasis on hygiene and cleanliness that certainly started to reduce the incidence of disease. Then, as a result of the industrial revolution, food supply improved, and in consequence people started to eat better and to live longer. In recent years there has been less loss of life due to war.

However, people do take time to adapt to a lower death rate. They won't realize immediately that more of their children will survive under the newly created improved living conditions. Thus although death rates fall there is a short gap before birth rates start falling, during which time the total population spurts forward.

In the industrialized countries, the fall in birth rate has occurred and so population increase has now dropped to a much slower rate than immediately after the effects of the improved living conditions were felt.

The situation in the underdeveloped countries is very different and somewhat more worrying. They have only recently experienced a great decrease in death rate, and it has been brought upon them very suddenly; the industrialized world has supplied them with medicines and insecticides to destroy disease-carrying insects and thus the death rate has been drastically reduced almost overnight. But the birth rate is as high as ever, for many of these people are not well educated, and it will take them some time to realize that they don't need to have about ten children in order to ensure that at least one or two will survive till adulthood – and it is important for them to have grown-up children, because each extra human being means another source of desperately needed income.

Population control

The more people there are on this earth the less room there is to grow food, and the 'eating-up' of the countryside is not a slow event. It is inevitable that with more people to house, urban areas will gradually extend into what was once lush, green, countryside.

We are also running out of natural resources; the one that immediately springs to mind is energy, the very item which makes the whole of the technological world tick, and remember we rely upon that world to keep food supplies high.

The need for population control is indeed enormous, and the heart of the problem lies in the vast regions of Latin America and parts of the Far East, Middle East and Africa. So far efforts to control population in these countries have been very unsuccessful. For instance, when they tried to introduce the pill as a form of birth control most attempts met with almost complete failure. These poorly educated women just cannot understand the importance of taking a pill each day in order to achieve total protection and anyway some don't even want that protection. Clearly, implementing a successful programme is not simply a matter of introducing tried and tested methods of Western control. A different approach is needed which has yet to be found.

Developing countries

Let me just put the problem of population increase to one side and take a look at another aspect of the situation.

At this moment in time you and I are all right, thank you very much; we have plenty to eat. This hasn't always been the case. We have had our fair share of famines in the past despite having fewer mouths to feed. Why is this so? Well, the simple answer is that in those days we had to rely greatly on locally grown food because there was no means of long-distance transport. If we happened to have a bad crop one year, which wasn't such an unusual event because there were no technological aids in those days to help the plants we grew through bad times, then we went without. We could not even rely on the excessively good years to help us out because there was no effective means of storing surplus. Grain kept from a good harvest, for instance, would soon be attacked by rats and mice, an event which can largely be overcome these days.

Thus the meteoric rise of technology for about one quarter of the world's population has meant that the possibility of starvation has been completely stamped out (for the time being at least), and in its place is the opportunity not only to feed adequately but also to feed upon a wide variety of different foods.

Technology and the accompanying wealth has by no means hit all parts of the globe; about three-quarters of the world's population is still living from crop to crop, very much as we once did, and often people die from starvation in these parts. An obvious example of this is Biafra, whose problems were highlighted during their recent civil war; and while each of us sat glued to a television set eating our supper, we saw heart-rending pictures of emaciated Biafrans literally dying from starvation before our very eyes.

We are aware of the problem, but the trouble is it is so far away from most of us that we tend to put it to the back of our minds. But there are people from the developed countries who devote all their energies to helping the underfed.

The Food and Agriculture Organization

This is an organization which was set up by the United Nations after the end of the Second World War. Its aim is to improve the nutrition of those from the underdeveloped world, and in order to achieve this 'objective' its attack must be wide-ranging.

First of all, it is necessary to understand the scope of the problem. They must find out how many people are under-nourished in each of the different areas, from which deficiency diseases they are suffering, and what natural resources they have at their disposal. Only after establishing these basic facts will anyone be able to offer a possible solution.

The FAO also promotes scientific, technical, social and economic research which is related to nutrition, food and agriculture. It also supports and organizes the teaching of proper infant feeding practices, which will hopefully reduce child mortality, and the teaching of nutrition, which will hopefully put an end to the many strange taboos and food habits to which many of these people cling.

For instance, if you take a look at a picture of an Indian village it is quite likely that you will see one or two cows wandering around completely free. The Indian people, due to their religious beliefs, consider all cows to be sacred and must, in consequence, never be used as a source of food. Obviously this taboo denies the Indian people of a very valuable source of nourishment, in particular, protein.

In Ethiopia ground-nuts, which are also a good source of protein, are thought to cause stillbirths. Thus women, who most need the valuable protein because of their large number of pregnancies are avoiding it because they mistakenly believe that more of their children will live if they don't eat this foodstuff.

There are many other seemingly nonsensical but firmly held beliefs which I could give you, and each one helps to aggravate the state of poor nutrition just that little bit more.

The FAO believes, quite rightly, that the immense improve-ments from the West in feeding people can be reproduced for the less privileged people of our present world; it is possible for them all to be fed better and thus to live healthier and happier lives.

There are other organizations who help to improve feeding in the underdeveloped world; two that immediately spring to mind and which you may have come across are WHO (the World Health Organization) and UNICEF (the United Nations International Children's Emergency Fund).

So you can see that although the problem of a food shortage

for you is a distant possibility due to the slow but steady increase in population and gradual dwindling of natural resources, it is very much a present-day reality for the people of the Third World who have a far larger population problem, together with a much lower rate of food production and poorer feeding practices.

Besides helping the underdeveloped nations to overcome their immediate food problems we must also think of our own future. I have explained above how a food shortage could be a distant possibility for us, and we must therefore continue to concentrate our efforts on increasing our own food supply as well as that of the developing nations, with the aim of ensuring adequate nutrition for all people of the world.

So let me now take a look at the ways we can increase our production of food and, indeed, the production of food in the underdeveloped countries, since it will ultimately affect what you – or should I say your children – will eat.

There are three main lines of attack open to us:

1. Improving the conventional food supply;
2. Making greater use of the more economical foods;
3. Using unconventional forms of food.

Improving the conventional food supply

Available land

First of all, it is worth considering how much more land there is available to produce food. Are we using all sources available to us? After all, Malthus was proved slightly wrong in his prediction because he failed to foresee that new farm land would be formed in such places as America and Australia. Are there more great expanses of earth 'waiting to be discovered' by the farmer? It would be fair to say that there aren't any that are readily available, but there is land which could be manipulated. Take, for example, a desert. Not exactly the kind of place where you would expect to see food being grown, but with the correct, albeit expensive, treatment a desert could be transformed into highly productive land; the same goes for forests and jungles. In our own country, where each year nearly 60000 acres are needed for urban housing, factories and recreation, careful planning could mean that only twenty per cent of this land need eat into agricultural parts; the rest can come from the derelict and waste land of the urban areas.

The sea, or rather lack of it, is another means of forming cultivatable land. The obvious example of this is the Zuider Zee project in Holland in which a quite sizeable amount of land was drained of sea water and is now used to grow food and provide space for housing.

In all it would be fair to say that we could, if we used every means available to us, double the amount of cultivatable land that we have at the moment.

It is, however, now possible to grow conventional food without the use of soil at all and instead by means of hydroponics! Let me explain. If you wanted to grow a lettuce, for example, you would place the seed in a long channel, and it would be constantly bathed by a continuous flow of water, minerals and carbon dioxide. With these basic chemicals your lettuce seed would be transformed into a lush green vegetable in a relatively short space of time. This technique has the advantage of avoiding disease because no spoilage organisms are present in the system. It can also produce substantially more crops each year than is possible by more conventional means. However, it is expensive and, of course, it will cover areas of land which might otherwise have been cultivated, although I do believe that this method of plant growth has gone under the ground in the Arctic. It may be that we shall be seeing more of it in the future.

Supplies from the sea

We also get food from the sea. But can supplies be increased from this source by improved methods of fishing, for instance? No doubt you are aware that our so-called staple diet of fish and chips is no longer so readily available. It pretty well priced itself out of the market during 1976. The chips went up because there was a shortage of potatoes due to a bad crop the year before, the fish went up for slightly more serious reasons. Some areas off the English coast have just been so well hunted that the amount of fish available to be caught is dwindling. So however much the fishing gear may be improved, it could all be in vain because there just isn't the fish to catch.

That is the case off the well-fished shores of England; there are, however, other parts of the world where there must surely be a largely untapped source of fodder under the water, and this undoubtedly could make a valuable contribution to the world food supplies.

Raising the amount of fish available in the sea by fertilizing, thus increasing the food they can eat, has been tried but it is not in commercial use anywhere due to its high cost; it has been found better to produce fish in specially prepared ponds. This is used to good effect in such countries as Malaysia and Israel, and it could undoubtedly be a useful way to increase the amount of available food.

Chemical improvers

For some time now crop yields have been greatly increased by means of fertilizers which help to feed the plants, and improved animal nutrition has meant greater yields in this area of production.

There are also other chemicals which are used to raise production, such as insecticides and herbicides on plants. The application of these two vastly increases supplies; the former kills off insects and other animals which might decide to make a meal of the crops before we have a look in, and the latter kills off any weeds which, if present in the soil, would undoubtedly adversely affect the growth of crops. Animals, too, are subjected to somewhat similar chemical invasions; for instance, antibiotics are given to counteract illness and infection which could adversely affect growth.

Of course, all these chemicals must be strictly controlled by law in much the same way as additives are carefully investigated, and even then some would say that they are not really desirable, but if you and I are to continue having enough to eat, they are a must.

Breeding the best

We have all been built in our own special way, and it is usual for us to reflect the shape of our parents – a point we can now understand due to the science of genetics. In much the same way plants and other animals are never identical to each other.

They have their own special characteristics, and this fact can and is used to advantage when it comes to increasing food production.

Much effort is put into breeding plants and animals that offer the best yields in the most economical fashion; this has been carried out since time immemorial but recently, with the understanding of why it all happens being made available to us, the whole process has been greatly advanced.

Most of this breeding has taken place in the developed world, but one or two significant improvements have been made in the underdeveloped world, improvements which caused what is now known as the Green Revolution. For instance, Mexico can now produce enough wheat and maize to feed its whole population, something which a few decades ago would have been totally unthinkable. The same has happened in the Philippines; they are now self-sufficient in rice.

As with all revolutions this one has caused society to turn upside down, and the political decisions which must now be faced are very great; for instance, many of the smaller farmers who are unable to afford the high prices being asked for fertilizers and who, in consequence, cannot make a living from the land, are drifting into the slums of the large cities – jobless and homeless. The ones that do stay on the land are doing just a little too well out of the situation.

Mass mechanization

You would be unlikely to find oxen pulling a plough anywhere in England these days. It is now the age of the tractor and of many other highly mechanical aids, all of which play their part in increasing food production.

As yet these mechanical monsters have not really arrived in the underdeveloped world, but moves are being made in this direction. For instance, the scythe has been introduced instead of the sickle in Ethiopia, which means that a farmer can now cut a good deal more of his crop at harvest time.

Irrigation

Water is the spring of life for plants and animals, and constantly newer and more efficient methods are being sought to improve supplies to areas in need. This is of particular relevance to the underdeveloped lands, which are very often areas of low rainfall.

Greater use of the more economical foods

Whenever you eat something, before it is eventually turned into muscle or fat or whatever, a fair amount is lost, either because it was unabsorbed in the first place or because it was used to fuel the chemical processes within your body.

Food from a primary source, such as vegetable and fruit, is not efficiently converted by an animal, and thus if you eat the latter, which is called a secondary source of food, it will undoubtedly have been less economic to produce than a primary source of food. This point can be most effectively illustrated by comparing the amount of land needed to produce so many calories or so much protein from the different food sources.

Take calories first of all. If you needed, say, 1000 Calories worth of energy, the amount of land that would be required to provide that amount of fuel from beef would be ten times that needed for wheat and twenty times that needed for potatoes. But are things any better for protein? After all, animals are always considered to be such a good source of this nutrient. I am afraid not. For instance, legumes such as beans need between ten and twenty-four times less space to produce the same amount of protein as beef cattle.

However, animals are prepared to eat grass and we are not, so the above figures should really be slightly readjusted. There is another very important consideration to be made about animals: we like eating them, and as you saw in Chapter 2 palatability is a very important part of good nutrition, so perhaps there is a limit to the amount of primary foods we are prepared to eat.

Unconventional forms of food

For some time now there has been a fairly widely held belief that the chief problem facing our diet is lack of protein, and for this reason research into 'new' foods, which I shall shortly tell you about, has been preoccupied with devising those that are rich sources of protein. Whether this is such a good idea for helping to feed the people of the world, particularly those in the under-developed nations, is debatable for what they now appear to need is calories (i.e. just more food in general) rather than protein.

We have perhaps been slightly misled into thinking that the latter nutrient is short, because distribution within the family is not always as it should be; for instance, there is a widespread belief that babies in the Third World who are most in need can survive on non-nutritious starchy foods whereas adults should have the more proteinous items. As a result kwashiorkor − a childhood disease caused by a shortage of protein in the diet − is widespread. In this case what is really required to put things right is education rather than protein and, perhaps, a general increase in the total amount of food that is available.

However, in spite of the changing attitude outlined above much research has already been carried out into finding accep-table 'new' forms of proteinous food which are economic in terms of space to produce, and we shall probably be made aware of the results before too long.

Textured Vegetable Protein (or TVP for short)

For many years that very nutritious food, the soya bean − and, indeed, other beans − have been used mainly as a source of animal foodstuff, but things are changing and the manufacturer is now employing his skills to transform this food into a product which closely resembles meat (it can also be used as a basis for other foods; I've even eaten chocolate truffles made partly from TVP!) and can, therefore, be enjoyed by us.

Basically, there are two production methods used. One is by extrusion, which is somewhat similar to the way spaghetti is produced by squeezing the mixture through nozzles, and the other method is by spinning, which is rather like the way nylon yarn is knitted to make tights. The end result of both techniques can be either chunks or granules of TVP.

At present you can buy TVP in one of two forms: either made up in the form of a conventional dish such as a stew or curry (it's usually partially mixed with ordinary meat which helps to mask the rather beany flavour), or in its 'pure' form as chunks or granules.

TVP is a good deal cheaper than normal meat and, in terms of land needed, is far more economical to produce. It is for your purposes as nutritious as meat, and it is already being used on a fairly large scale in school lunches because of its low cost. The children seem to quite like it, too.

The main reason why TVP on its own doesn't taste the same (and some say as good) as ordinary meat is because it has a very much lower fat content, which means its calorie value is a good deal less. But as soon as it is added to meat it absorbs fat very easily which cancels out this difference.

TVP on its own is a boon for the man on the coronary risk list. It is very low in saturated fat and contains virtually no cholesterol.

I feel certain that you shall be seeing more of this effective little meat substitute, particularly when it starts appearing in quantity in general food stores rather than just health food shops, which appears to be the case at the moment.

Green leaves

Another very much less familiar (although familiar in its 'natural' form) food is the protein from green leaves. Actually you can't buy this in the shops like you can soya protein because so far when it has been tested out on us we have tended to turn up our noses at it; but one day it may well be made into an acceptable form.

The tough fibrous material which is left after the proteinous juice has been removed has found a role as a form of food for animals (such as the cow) which can make use of this type of sustenance. So if the proteinous juice can be fed to animals which can't make use of fibrous materials, the development of the leaf as a form of food for animals could, at least, become an economic proposition.

Micro-organisms

Several companies have been investigating the possibility of growing micro-organisms on a large scale as a protein source.

These include bacteria, which contain anything up to about ninety per cent of their dry weight as protein; yeast, which contains about fifty per cent; and fungi and algae, which each contain about forty per cent. They only need a very limited amount of space in order to be produced, but their use as a human foodstuff is still some way off, if ever, because their effects once within the human body may not be wholly desirable and they are still very expensive to produce.

Non-foods

Work is being carried out to see whether we can obtain protein from wool and carbohydrate from wood. Who knows; before long we may be eating woollen soup and sugared wood!

Sharing what we've got

So you see, we can produce enough food and, indeed, enough for future generations, but that still doesn't definitely mean that our aim – to feed all – will be met, because so often food is poorly distributed. It may be that it never reaches its destination, due to poor roads or lack of preservation; it may be that there is an unfair share-out within the family, with the children going without their much needed protein; it may be that the poor can't afford the more nutritious food. These are just a few of the problems which hamper proper distribution, and they must be as actively fought against as population increase and inadequate food production if we are ever to achieve and maintain our aim of healthy eating for all.

Appendices

Appendix A

Energy and nutrient chart

Points to Note:

1 Nearly all the values given here are based upon those found in the McCance and Widdowson food tables (*The Composition of Foods*, H M S O , 1969).

2 The joule value is always calculated by multiplying the calorie value by 4.2.

3 One carbohydrate unit represents 5 g. of carbohydrate. Some tables equate one unit with 10 g. of carbohydrate, in which case their units would be equal to half the ones you can see in this list.

All units are given to the nearest $\frac{1}{2}$ (neg. indicates that a food contains less than a $\frac{1}{4}$ of a unit but more than 0).

4 If a food or drink is a good source of the chief nutrients (i.e. protein, fat, carbohydrate, alcohol, calcium, iron, vitamins A, B1, B2, nicotinic acid, C and D) then that nutrient will be listed in the column entitled 'Which Nutrients?'

5 A food has been classified as a good source of a particular nutrient by taking into account both the amount of a certain nutrient it contains and also the normal portion size. For instance, although potatoes per ounce don't always contain that much vitamin C they can be considered as a good source of this nutrient because they are normally eaten in quite large amounts, thus the intake of vitamin C overall is quite high.

It is true that this form of classification is rather a matter of personal judgement, but the aim is to provide you with a guide that is both practical and easy to follow without confusing the issue with too many numbers.

6 All the food items and milk are dealt with in the first group which is called 'FOOD GROUP'; all the remaining drinks are dealt with in the second group which is called 'DRINK GROUP'.

7   Carbohydrate units for drinks containing alcohol are measured in carbohydrate unit equivalents; any alcohol present having been treated as carbohydrate on a calorie for calorie basis. This is because alcoholic drinks must be restricted if a low-carbohydrate slimming regime is to work.

Food Group

Food	Amount*	Calorie value	Kilojoule value	Carbohydrate units	Which nutrients?
Almonds – shelled, raw	1 oz.	170	714	neg	Protein, fat, iron
Anchovies (6 fillets)	1 oz.	40	168	0	—
Apples – flesh only	1 oz.	13	55	½	Carbohydrate
average-sized fruit	4 oz.	40	168	2	
Apricots – fresh (with stone)	1 oz.	7	29	½	—
– canned in syrup	1 oz.	30	126	1½	Carbohydrate and iron – for dried apricots only
– dried	1 oz.	52	218	2½	
Arrowroot	1 oz.	100	420	5½	Carbohydrate
Artichokes – globe, boiled (as served)	1 oz.	2	8	neg	—
– Jerusalem, boiled	1 oz.	5	21	neg	—
Asparagus – boiled	1 oz.	5	21	neg	Vitamin C
Aubergines – raw	1 oz.	4	17	neg	Vitamin C
Avocado pears – flesh only	1 oz.	63	265	neg	Vitamin C, and it is unusually high in fat for a fruit
Bacon – back, raw	1 oz.	121	508	0	Protein, fat, Vitamin B1
– streaky, raw	1 oz.	115	483	0	
Bananas – with skin	1 oz.	13	55	½	Carbohydrate
– average-sized fruit	6 oz.	78	328	4	
Barley – raw	1 oz.	102	428	4½	Carbohydrate
– boiled	1 oz.	34	143	1½	

*1 oz. = 25 g.   1 fl. oz. = 30 ml.   1 pint = 600 ml.

Food Group—contd.

Food	Amount	Calorie value	Kilojoule value	Carbohydrate units	Which nutrients?
Bass — steamed (+bone)	1 oz.	19	80	0	Protein
Beans — baked	1 oz.	26	109	1	Protein, carbohydrate
— broad, boiled	1 oz.	12	50	$\frac{1}{2}$	Protein, carbohydrate, vitamin C
— butter, boiled	1 oz.	26	109	1	Protein, carbohydrate
— haricot, boiled	1 oz.	25	105	1	Protein, carbohydrate
— runner, boiled	1 oz.	2	8	neg	Vitamin C
— french, boiled	1 oz.	2	8	neg	Vitamin C
Beef — steak, grilled	1 oz.	48	202	0	Protein, iron, vitamin B2, nicotinic acid
— sirloin, roast, lean only	1 oz.	64	269	0	
— corned	1 oz.	64	277	0	
Beetroot — boiled	1 oz.	13	55	$\frac{1}{2}$	Vitamin C
Biscuits — plain	1 oz.	122	512	4	
— sweet	1 oz.	140	588	4	Fat, carbohydrate
— chocolate	1 oz.	141	592	4	
Blackberries — raw	1 oz.	8	34	$\frac{1}{2}$	Vitamin C
Blackcurrants — raw	1 oz.	8	34	$\frac{1}{2}$	Vitamin C
Bloaters — grilled, without bone and skin	1 oz.	73	307	0	Protein, vitamins A, B1, D and nicotinic acid
Brains — boiled	1 oz.	30	126	0	Protein, vitamins B1, B2 and nicotinic acid
Bran	1 oz.	58	244	$1\frac{1}{2}$	Carbohydrate

Food	Measure				Chief nutrients
Brazil nuts – shelled	1 oz.	183	769	neg	Protein, fat
Bread – white or brown	1 oz.	70	294	3	Protein, carbohydrate, calcium, iron, vitamins, B1 and nicotinic acid
Breakfast cereals – e.g. cornflakes	1 oz.	104	437	5	Carbohydrate, iron and due to additions, vitamins B1, B2 and nicotinic acid
Broccoli – boiled	1 oz.	4	17	neg	Vitamin C
Brussels sprouts – boiled	1 oz.	5	21	neg	Vitamin C
Butter	1 oz.	226	949	neg	Fat, vitamins A and D
Cabbage – red or white, raw	1 oz.	7	29	neg	Vitamin C
– red or white, boiled	1 oz.	3	13	neg	
Cake – plain	1 oz.	121	508	3	Fat, carbohydrate
– rich fruit	1 oz.	104	437	3	
Carrots –raw	1 oz.	6	25	½	Vitamin A
–boiled	1 oz.	5	21	neg	
Cauliflower – raw	1 oz.	7	29	neg	Vitamin C
– boiled	1 oz.	3	13	neg	
Celery – raw	1 oz.	3	13	neg	—
Cheese – hard e.g. Cheddar	1 oz.	120	504	neg	Protein fat, vitamins A and B2
– cream	1 oz.	232	974	neg	Fat, vitamin A
– cottage	1 oz.	32	134	neg	Protein
Cherries – with stones	1 oz.	11	40	1	—
Chestnuts – flesh only	1 oz.	49	206	2	Carbohydrate
Chicken – meat only, raw	1 oz.	33	139	0	Protein and nicotinic acid
– meat only, roast	1 oz.	54	227	0	

Food Group—contd.

Food	Amount	Calorie value	Kilojoule value	Carbohydrate units	Which nutrients?
Chicory – raw	1 oz.	3	13	neg	Vitamin C
Chives – raw	1 oz.	8	34	neg	—
Chocolate – milk	1 oz.	167	701	3	Fat, carbohydrate
– plain	1 oz.	155	651	3	
Chutney – apple	1 oz.	55	231	3	Carbohydrate
Cocoa powder	1 oz.	128	538	2	Carbohydrate, iron
Coconut – fresh, flesh	1 oz.	104	437	neg	Fat
– desiccated	1 oz.	178	748	$\frac{1}{2}$	Fat
Cod – raw, fillet	1 oz.	22	92	0	Protein
Codliver oil	1 oz.	264	1109	0	Fat, vitamins A and D
Cod roe – raw	1 oz.	37	155	0	Protein, fat, vitamins B1 and B2
Corn oil	1 oz.	260	1092	0	Fat
Corn on the cob – raw	1 oz.	28	118	1	Carbohydrate
Cornflour	1 oz.	100	420	5	Carbohydrate
Courgettes – raw	1 oz.	2	8	neg	—
Crab – meat only, boiled	1 oz.	36	151	0	Protein, vitamins B1 and nicotinic acid
Cranberries – raw	1 oz.	4	17	neg	Vitamin C
Cranberry Sauce	1 oz.	43	181	$2\frac{1}{2}$	Carbohydrate
Cream – double	1 oz.	131	550	neg	
– single	1 oz.	62	260	neg	
– clotted	1 oz.	164	689	neg	Fat, vitamin A
– soured	1 oz.	54	227	neg	

Food	Quantity				Constituents
Cucumber – raw	1 oz.	3	13	neg	—
Currants – dried	1 oz.	69	290	3½	Carbohydrate
Custard powder	1 oz.	100	420	5	Carbohydrate
Damsons – raw, with stones	1 oz.	9	38	½	—
Dates – with stones	1 oz.	61	256	3	Carbohydrate
Dripping – from beef	1 oz.	262	1100	0	Fat
Duck – meat only, roast	1 oz.	89	374	0	Protein, fat
Dumpling	1 oz.	59	248	1½	Carbohydrate
Eel – meat only, cooked	1 oz.	106	445	0	Protein, fat, vitamins A and D
Eggs – white, raw	1 oz.	11	46	neg	—
– yolk, raw	1 oz.	99	416	neg	Protein, fat, iron, vitamins A, B2 and D
– whole egg, standard, raw	2 oz.	80	336	neg	
Figs – fresh	1 oz.	12	50	½	—
– dried, raw	1 oz.	61	256	3	Carbohydrate, iron
Flounder – on bone, steamed	1 oz.	15	63	0	Protein
Flour – white, enriched	1 oz.	100	420	5	Protein, carbohydrate, calcium, iron, vitamin B1 and nicotinic acid
– soya, full fat	1 oz.	123	517	1	
Garlic	1 clove	2	8	neg	—
Gelatin powder	1 oz.	70	294	0	Protein, fat
Goose – roast, meat only	1 oz.	92	386	0	Protein, fat
Gooseberries – ripe	1 oz.	10	42	½	Vitamin C
Grapefruit – flesh only	1 oz.	6	25	½	Vitamin C
Grapes – whole, black or white	1 oz.	15	63	1	
Greengages – fresh, with stones	1 oz.	13	55	½	
Grouse – roast, meat only	1 oz.	49	206	0	Protein, iron
Guinea fowl – roast, meat only	1 oz.	60	252	0	Protein, iron

Food Group—contd.

Food	Amount	Calorie value	Kilojoule value	Carbohydrate units	Which nutrients?
Haddock – fillet, white, raw	1 oz.	20	84	0	Protein
– fillet, smoked, raw	1 oz.	28	118	0	Protein
Hake – fillet, raw	1 oz.	21	88	0	Protein
Halibut – fillet, raw	1 oz.	41	172	0	Protein
Ham – lean only, boiled	1 oz.	62	260	0	Protein, nicotinic acid
Heart – lamb's, raw	1 oz.	45	189	0	Protein, iron, nicotinic acid
Herring – fillet, raw	1 oz.	67	281	0	Protein, fat, vitamin D and nicotinic acid
Honey	1 oz.	82	344	$4\frac{1}{2}$	Carbohydrate
Horseradish sauce	1 oz.	10	42	neg	—
Ice Cream – vanilla	1 oz.	55	231	1	Carbohydrate
Icing – glacé	1 oz.	105	441	5	Carbohydrate
Jam	1 oz.	74	312	4	Carbohydrate
Jelly cubes	1 oz.	75	315	$3\frac{1}{2}$	Carbohydrate
Kidney – raw, any kind	1 oz.	34	143	0	Protein, vitamins A, B1 and nicotinic acid
Kippers – flesh only, baked	1 oz.	57	239	0	Protein, fat, nicotinic acid
Lamb – roast, lean only	1 oz.	83	349	0	Protein, iron, nicotinic acid
Lard	1 oz.	262	1100	0	Fat
Leeks – raw	1 oz.	9	38	$\frac{1}{2}$	Vitamin C
Lemon – with skin	1 oz.	4	17	neg	Vitamin C
Lemon juice	1 fl. oz.	2	8	neg	Vitamin C
Lentils – raw	1 oz.	84	353	3	Protein, carbohydrate, iron, vitamins B1 and nicotinic acid

Food	Quantity				Chief nutrients
Lettuce – raw	1 oz.	3	13	neg	Vitamin C
Liver – lamb's, raw	1 oz.	36	151	0	Protein, iron, vitamins A, B2, C, D and nicotinic acid
Lobster – boiled, with shell	1 oz.	12	50	0	Protein
– boiled, flesh only	1 oz.	34	143	0	
Loganberries – raw	1 oz.	5	21	neg	Vitamin C
Luncheon meat	1 oz.	95	399	1	Protein, fat, nicotinic acid
Macaroni – raw	1 oz.	102	428	4½	Carbohydrate
– boiled	1 oz.	32	134	1½	
Mackerel – fried, on bone	1 oz.	39	164	0	Protein, vitamins A and D
Mandarins – with skin	1 oz.	7	29	neg	Vitamin C
Margarine	1 oz.	226	949	neg	Fat, vitamins A and D
low-fat spread	1 oz.	104	437	0	
Marmalade	1 oz.	74	311	4	Carbohydrate
Marrow – boiled	1 oz.	2	8	neg	—
Marzipan	1 oz.	124	521	4	Carbohydrate
Melon – cantaloupe and yellow with skin	1 oz.	4	17	neg	Vitamin C
– water melon, with skin	1 oz.	13	3	neg	
Milk – whole	1 pint	370	1554	5½	Protein, fat, carbohydrate, calcium, vitamins, A, B1, B2 and nicotinic acid
– separated	1 pint	200	840	5½	All the nutrients mentioned above except for fat and vitamin A
– made from reconstituted low-fat powdered milk	1 pint	200	849	5½	
Mincemeat	1 oz.	37	155	1½	Carbohydrate
Mint – raw	1 oz.	2	8	neg	—
Mullet – flesh only, steamed	1 oz.	36	151	0	Protein

Food Group—contd.

Food	Amount	Calorie value	Kilojoule value	Carbohydrate units	Which nutrients?
Mushrooms – raw	1 oz.	2	8	0	—
Mussels – boiled, with shells	1 oz.	7	29	neg	Iron
Mustard and cress	1 oz.	3	13	neg	Vitamin C
Mustard – made up	1 tsp	17	71	neg	—
Noodles – cooked	1 oz.	35	147	1½	Carbohydrate
Oatmeal	1 oz.	115	483	4	Carbohydrate, iron, vitamin B1
Olive oil	1 oz.	264	1109	0	Fat
Olives – with stone, in brine	1 oz.	24	101	neg	—
Onions – raw	1 oz.	7	29	½	Vitamin C
Oranges – raw, with skin	1 oz.	8	34	½	Vitamin C
Oysters – with shells, raw	1 oz.	2	8	neg	Iron
Parsley – raw	1 oz.	6	25	neg	Vitamin C
Parsnips – raw	1 oz.	14	59	½	Vitamin C
Pastry – baked, shortcrust	1 oz.	157	659	3	Fat, carbohydrate
– baked, flaky	1 oz.	167	701	2½	
Peaches – raw, with stones	1 oz.	9	38	½	—
Peanuts – roasted, shelled	1 oz.	171	718	½	Protein, fat, nicotinic acid
Peanut butter	1 oz.	176	739	½	
Pears – raw, eating, flesh only	1 oz.	12	50	½	
– 1 whole eating	4 oz.	36	151	1½	Carbohydrate
Peas – boiled	1 oz.	14	59	½	Carbohydrate, vitamin C
Peppers – red or green, raw	1 oz.	10	420	neg	Vitamin C

Food		Cal.	kJ	Carb.	Nutrients
Pheasant – roast, on bone	1 oz.	38	160	0	Protein, iron
Pigeon – roast, on bone	1 oz.	29	122	0	Protein, iron
Pilchards – canned, fish only	1 oz.	54	227	0	Protein, fat, calcium, iron
Pineapple – raw, flesh only	1 oz.	13	55	½	Carbohydrate
– canned in syrup	1 oz.	22	92	1	
Plaice – fillet, raw	1 oz.	22	92	0	Protein
– fillet, steamed	1 oz.	26	109	0	
Plums – dessert, raw with stones	1 oz.	10	42	½	Carbohydrate
Pork – roast	1 oz.	90	378	0	Protein, vitamins B1 and nicotinic acid
Porridge	1 oz.	13	55	½	Carbohydrate
Potatoes – boiled	1 oz.	23	97	1	Protein, carbohydrate, vitamins B1, C and nicotinic acid. Note that instant powder is only a good source of the vitamins B1 and C if they have been added by the manufacturer
– instant powder	1 oz.	105	441	4½	
– crisps	1 oz.	159	668	3	
– roast	1 oz.	32	134	1½	
– fried	1 oz.	68	286	2	
Prawns – without shells	1 oz.	30	126	0	Protein
Prunes – dried, no stones	1 oz.	38	160	2	Carbohydrate
– stewed, with stones	1 oz.	19	80	1	
Rabbit – on bone, stewed	1 oz.	26	109	0	Protein, iron, nicotinic acid
Radishes	1 oz.	4	17	neg	Vitamin C
Raisins	1 oz.	70	294	3½	Carbohydrate
Raspberries – raw	1 oz.	7	29	½	Vitamin C
Redcurrants – raw	1 oz.	6	25	neg	Vitamin C
Rhubarb – raw	1 oz.	2	8	neg	—

Food Group—contd.

Food	Amount	Calorie value	Kilojoule value	Carbohydrate units	Which nutrients?
Rice, white – raw	1 oz.	102	428	5	Carbohydrate
– boiled	1 oz.	35	147	$1\frac{1}{2}$	
Sago – raw	1 oz.	101	424	5	Carbohydrate
Salad cream	1 oz.	111	466	$\frac{1}{2}$	Fat
Salmon – steamed, whole fish	1 oz.	46	193	0	Protein, nicotinic acid
– canned	1 oz.	39	164	0	
– smoked	1 oz.	49	206	0	
Salt	1 oz.	0	0	0	—
Sardines – canned, fish only	1 oz.	84	353	0	Protein, fat, calcium, iron, vitamins B1 and nicotinic acid
Sausages – average, raw, pork	1 oz.	104	437	$\frac{1}{2}$	Protein, fat, vitamins B1 and nicotinic acid
Scallops – steamed	1 oz.	30	126	neg	Protein
Scampi – fried	1 oz.	60	252	neg	Protein, fat (due to frying)
Semolina – raw	1 oz.	100	420	$4\frac{1}{2}$	Carbohydrate
Shortbread	1 oz.	148	622	$3\frac{1}{2}$	Carbohydrate, fat
Shrimps – without shells	1 oz.	32	134	0	Protein
Snails – flesh only	1 oz.	26	109	neg	Protein
Sole – fillet, raw	1 oz.	22	92	0	Protein
Soup – thick, canned	$\frac{1}{2}$ pint	100–140	420–588	3–4	
– moderately thick, canned	$\frac{1}{2}$ pint	50–100	210–420	2–3	Carbohydrate
– clear, canned	$\frac{1}{2}$ pint	30–50	126–210	1–2	

Spaghetti – raw	1 oz.	104	437	5	
– boiled	1 oz.	32	134	1½	Carbohydrate
– canned in tomato sauce	1 oz.	17	71	½	
Spinach – boiled	1 oz.	7	29	neg	Vitamins A and C
Spring greens – boiled	1 oz.	3	13	neg	Vitamin C
Stock cube – Knorr	each	30	126	neg	—
Strawberries – raw	1 oz.	7	29	½	Vitamin C
Sturgeon – on bone, raw	1 oz.	27	113	0	Protein
Suet – block	1 oz.	262	1100	0	Fat
Sugar – white or brown	1 oz.	112	470	6	Carbohydrate
Sultanas	1 oz.	71	298	3½	Carbohydrate
Swedes – boiled	1 oz.	5	21	neg	Vitamin C
Sweetbreads – stewed	1 oz.	51	214	0	Protein
Sweetcorn – fresh or frozen, raw	1 oz.	28	118	1	—
Sweets – boiled	1 oz.	93	391	5	Carbohydrate
Syrups – golden	1 oz.	84	353	4½	Carbohydrate
– maple	1 oz.	71	298	4	Carbohydrate
– rosehip	1 oz.	70	294	3½	Carbohydrate, vitamin C
Tangerines – with skin	1 oz.	7	29	½	Vitamin C
Tapioca – raw	1 oz.	101	424	5½	Carbohydrate
Toffees	1 oz.	123	517	4	Carbohydrate
Tomatoes – raw	1 oz.	4	17	neg	Vitamin C
Tomato Ketchup	1 oz.	28	118	1½	Carbohydrate
Tongue – boiled	1 oz.	84	353	0	Protein, iron
Treacle – black	1 oz.	73	307	4	Carbohydrate, calcium, iron
Tripe – stewed	1 oz.	29	122	0	Protein
Trout – on bone, steamed	1 oz.	29	122	0	Protein
Tuna – canned in oil	1 oz.	84	353	0	Protein, fat

Food Group—contd.

Food	Amount	Calorie value	Kilojoule value	Carbohydrate units	Which nutrients?
Turbot – steamed	1 oz.	28	118	0	Protein
Turkey – meat only, roast	1 oz.	56	235	0	Protein, iron and nicotinic acid
Turnips – raw	1 oz.	5	21	neg	Vitamin C
Veal – fillet, raw	1 oz.	31	130	0	Protein, iron and nicotinic acid
– fillet, roast	1 oz.	66	277	0	
Venison – roast, meat only	1 oz.	56	235	0	Protein, iron and nicotinic acid
Vinegar	1 oz.	1	4	neg	—
Walnuts – flesh only	1 oz.	156	655	neg	Protein, fat
Watercress	1 oz.	4	17	neg	Vitamins A and C
Wheatgerm	1 oz.	101	424	3	Vitamin B1
Whitebait – fried	1 oz.	152	638	neg	Protein, fat, calcium, iron
Whiting – on bone, raw	1 oz.	12	50	0	Protein
Winkles – boiled, without shells	1 oz.	27	113	neg	Protein, iron
Yeast – fresh	1 oz.	15	63	neg	Vitamins B1, B2 and nicotinic acid
– dried	1 oz.	48	202	neg	
– extract, e.g. marmite	1 oz.	51	214	neg	
Yoghurt – natural	5 fl. oz.	100	420	2	Same as whole milk
– low fat, natural	5 fl. oz.	75	315	2	Same as separated milk
– fruit flavoured	5 fl. oz.	115	483	4	Both these contain similar nutrients to whole milk but are overall less nutritious because they have more carbohydrate at the expense of other nutrients
– whole fruit	5 fl. oz.	136	571	5	

(All are average values only)

Drinks Group

Drink	Amount	Calorie value	Kilojoule value	Carbohydrate units	Which nutrients?
Soft varieties					
(All these are average values only)					
American ginger ale – one small bottle	4 fl. oz.	40	168	2	Carbohydrate
Bitter lemon – one small bottle	4 fl. oz.	40	168	2	Carbohydrate
Blackcurrant – concentrated	1 fl. oz.	35	147	2	Carbohydrate
Coca-Cola – an average sized bottle	6½ fl. oz.	80	336	4	Carbohydrate
Dandelion and Burdock	1 fl. oz.	9	38	½	Carbohydrate
Dry ginger ale – one small bottle	4 fl. oz.	20	84	1	Carbohydrate
Ginger beer – one average bottle	6 fl. oz.	65	273	4	Carbohydrate
Grapefruit – concentrated	1 fl. oz.	30	126	1½	Carbohydrate
– juice, unsweetened	1 fl. oz.	11	46	½	
Lemon – juice, unsweetened	1 fl. oz.	13	55	½	
– concentrated	1 fl. oz.	30	126	1½	Carbohydrate
Lemonade – fizzy, one small bottle	4 fl. oz.	24	101	1½	Carbohydrate
Lime juice – concentrated	1 fl. oz.	32	134	2	Carbohydrate
Lucozade	1 fl. oz.	19	80	1	Carbohydrate

Drinks Group—contd.

Drink	Amount	Calorie value	Kilojoule value	Carbohydrate units	Which nutrients?
Low-calorie drinks	1 fl. oz.	less than 2	less than 8	0	—
Milk shakes — made up with milk	1 fl. oz.	25	105	$\frac{1}{2}$	Same as for whole milk
Mineral water	1 fl. oz.	0	0	0	—
Orange — concentrated	1 fl. oz.	39	164	2	
— juice, unsweetened	1 fl. oz.	11	46	$\frac{1}{2}$	Carbohydrate
— fizzy	1 fl. oz.	10	42	$\frac{1}{2}$	
Pineapple juice — one small bottle	4 fl. oz.	72	302	$3\frac{1}{2}$	Carbohydrate
Ribena — very sweet blackcurrant concentrate	1 fl. oz.	83	349	4	Carbohydrate, vitamin C
Tomato juice — one small bottle	4 fl. oz.	28	118	$1\frac{1}{2}$	Carbohydrate
Tonic water — one small bottle	4 fl. oz.	28	118	$1\frac{1}{2}$	Carbohydrate

(Note: only those drinks which specifically state that they contain vitamin C will be a source of this nutrient. Most are not.)

Alcoholic varieties

Drink	Amount	Calorie value	Kilojoule value	Carbohydrate units	Which nutrients?
Beer — brown ale	1 pint	160	672	8	
— draught bitter	1 pint	180	756	$8\frac{1}{2}$	
— draught mild	1 pint	140	588	7	Carbohydrate, nicotinic acid
— pale ale	1 pint	180	756	9	alcohol
— stout, bottled	1 pint	200	840	$10\frac{1}{2}$	
— stout, extra	1 pint	220	924	11	
— strong ale	1 pint	420	1764	20	

G

Brandy* – standard pub measure (⅙ gill)	⅙ of 5 fl. oz.	52	218	2½	Alcohol
Bourbon* – standard pub measure (⅙ gill)	⅙ of 5 fl. oz.	52	218	2½	Alcohol
Campari – standard pub measure (⅓ gill)	⅓ of 5 fl. oz.	115	483	6	Alcohol
Cider – dry	1 pint	200	840	10½	Carbohydrate, alcohol
– sweet	1 pint	240	1008	12	
– vintage	1 pint	400	1680	29	
Gin* – standard pub measure (⅙ gill)	⅙ of 5 fl. oz.	52	218	2½	Alcohol
Liqueurs – standard pub measure (⅙ gill), values vary according to type – usually the more syrupy they are the the higher the calorie and carbohydrate value	⅙ of 5 fl. oz.	60–100	252–420	3–5	Carbohydrate, alcohol
Port – ruby (⅓ gill)	⅓ of 5 fl. oz.	72	302	3½	Carbohydrate, alcohol
– tawny (⅓ gill)	⅓ of 5 fl. oz.	90	378	4	
Rum* – standard pub measure (⅙ gill)	⅙ of 5 fl. oz.	52	218	2½	Alcohol
Shandy Bass – bottled or canned	½ pint	60	252	4	Carbohydrate
Sherry – dry, standard pub measure (⅓ gill)	⅓ of 5 fl. oz.	55	231	2½	Carbohydrate
– sweet, standard pub measure (⅓ gill)	⅓ of 5 fl. oz.	63	265	3	Carbohydrate, alcohol

*All at 70° proof

Drinks Group—contd.

Drink	Amount	Calorie value	Kilojoule value	Equivalent carbohydrate units	Which nutrients?
Vermouth – dry, standard pub measure ($\frac{1}{3}$ gill)	$\frac{1}{3}$ of 5 fl. oz.	60	252	3	Carbohydrate, alcohol
Vermouth – sweet, standard pub measure ($\frac{1}{3}$ gill)	$\frac{1}{3}$ of 5 fl. oz.	80	336	4	Carbohydrate, alcohol
Vodka* – standard pub measure ($\frac{1}{6}$ gill)	$\frac{1}{6}$ of 5 fl. oz.	52	218	$2\frac{1}{2}$	Alcohol
Whisky* – standard pub measure ($\frac{1}{6}$ gill)	$\frac{1}{6}$ of 5 fl. oz.	52	218	$2\frac{1}{2}$	Alcohol
Wine – standard pub measure					
– Champagne	4 fl. oz.	84	353	4	Alcohol and for the sweet wines – carbohydrate
– Graves	4 fl. oz.	84	353	$4\frac{1}{2}$	
– Sauternes	4 fl. oz.	104	437	$5\frac{1}{2}$	
– Australian burgundy	4 fl. oz.	80	336	4	
– Beaujolais	4 fl. oz.	76	319	4	
– Chianti	4 fl. oz.	72	302	$3\frac{1}{2}$	
– Medoc	4 fl. oz.	72	302	$3\frac{1}{2}$	

*All at 70° proof

Appendix B

The Department of Health and Social Security's recommended calorie and nutrient intakes, 1969

Age ranges (a)		Energy (c)		Recommended	Protein Minimum requirement	Calcium
years		MJ (d)	kcal	g (e)	g	mg
Infants						
Under 1 (b)		3.3	800	20	15	600
Children						
1		5.0	1200	30	19	500
2		5.9	1400	35	21	500
3–4		6.7	1600	40	25	500
5–6		7.5	1800	45	28	500
7–8		8.8	2100	53	30	500
Males						
9–11		10.5	2500	63	36	700
12–14		11.7	2800	70	46	700
15–17		12.6	3000	75	50	600
18–34	sedentary	11.3	2700	68	45	500
	moderately active	12.6	3000	75	45	500
	very active	15.1	3600	90	45	500
35–64	sedentary	10.9	2600	65	43	500
	moderately active	12.1	2900	73	43	500
	very active	15.1	3600	90	43	500
65–74		9.8	2350	59	39	500
75 and over		8.8	2100	53	38	500
Females						
9–11		9.6	2300	58	35	700
12–14		9.6	2300	58	44	700
15–17		9.6	2300	58	40	600
18–54	most occupations	9.2	2200	55	38	500
	very active	10.5	2500	63	38	500
55–74		8.6	2050	51	36	500
75 and over		8.0	1900	48	34	500
Pregnant, 2nd and 3rd trimesters		10.0	2400	60	44	1200 (l)
Lactating		11.3	2700	68	55	1200

(a) The ages are from one birthday to another: e.g. 9 up to 12 is from the 9th up to but not including the 12th birthday. The figures in the Table in general refer to the mid-point of the ranges though those for the range 18 up to 34 refer to the age 25 years and for the range 18 up to 54 to 35 years of age.

(b) Average figures relating to the first year of life. Energy and minimum protein requirements for the four trimesters are given elsewhere in the DHSS report.

(c) Average requirements relating to groups of individuals.

(d) Megajoules (10⁶ joules). Calculated from the relation 1 kilocalorie 4.186 kilojoules, and rounded to 1 decimal place.

(e) Recommended intakes calculated as providing 10 per cent of energy requirements.

(f) The figures, calculated from energy requirements and the recommended intake of thiamin of 0.4 mg/1000 kcal, relate to groups of individuals.

Iron mg	Vitamin A (retinol equivalent) μg (h)	Thiamin mg (f)	Riboflavin mg	Nicotinic acid equivalent mg (g)	Vitamin C mg	Vitamin D μg (i)
6 (k)	450	0.3	0.4	5	15	10
7	300	0.5	0.6	7	20	10
7	300	0.6	0.7	8	20	10
8	300	0.6	0.8	9	20	10
8	300	0.7	0.9	10	20	2.5
10	400	0.8	1.0	11	20	2.5
13	575	1.0	1.2	14	25	2.5
14	725	1.1	1.4	16	25	2.5
15	750	1.2	1.7	19	30	2.5
10	750	1.1	1.7	18	30	2.5
10	750	1.2	1.7	18	30	2.5
10	750	1.4	1.7	18	30	2.5
10	750	1.0	1.7	18	30	2.5
10	750	1.2	1.7	18	30	2.5
10	750	1.4	1.7	18	30	2.5
10	750	0.9	1.7	18	30	2.5
10	750	0.8	1.7	18	30	2.5
13	575	0.9	1.2	13	25	2.5
14	725	0.9	1.4	16	25	2.5
15	750	0.9	1.4	16	30	2.5
12	750	0.9	1.3	15	30	2.5
12	750	1.0	1.3	15	30	2.5
10	750	0.8	1.3	15	30	2.5
10	750	0.7	1.3	15	30	2.5
15	750	1.0	1.6	18	60	10 (j)
15	1200	1.1	1.8	21	60	10

(g) 1 nicotinic acid equivalent = 1 mg available nicotinic acid or 60 mg tryptophan.
(h) 1 retinol equivalent = 1 μg retinol or 6 μg β-carotene or 12 μg other biologically carotenoids.
(i) No dietary source may be necessary for those adequately exposed to sunlight, but the requirement for the housebound may be greater than that recommended.
(j) For all three trimesters.
(k) These figures apply to infants who are not breast fed. Infants who are entirely breast fed receive smaller quantities; these are adequate since absorption from breast milk is higher.
(l) For the third trimester only.

Appendix C

Slimming Diets

Two types of slimming diets are shown here:

1 Calorie-controlled.
2 Carbohydrate-controlled.

Calorie – controlled

The calorie breakdown of this diet is as follows:

Basic Diet (Approximately 1000 Calories)

Meal	Approximate Calorie Value
Breakfast	150
Lunch	250
Dinner	350

Daily Allowances

300 ml. (½ pint) of milk	185
6 g. (¼ oz.) of butter or margarine	55
Vegetables from free allowance	10
Total	1000

Each extra is approximately 250 Calories and may either be included with a meal or as a separate snack.

Guidelines for the diet

1 Choose one breakfast, one lunch and one dinner each day. It doesn't matter if you wish to swop the lunch and dinner around, i.e. have your main meal at midday and your light meal in the evening.
2 Each day allow yourself 6 g. (¼ oz.) of butter or margarine, or 12 g. (½ oz.) of a low-fat spread, and 300 ml. (½ pint) of whole milk or 600 ml. (1 pint) of low-fat milk.

3   Depending upon the amount of weight you have to lose and upon your sex you may increase your daily calorie intake above the basic allowance of 1000 Calories by choosing from the daily extra list at the end of the diet.
4   You may have as much tea and coffee as you like so long as you don't use more than 300 ml. (½ pint) of whole milk and so long as you use artificial sweeteners instead of sugar.
All low-calorie drinks can be taken without any restriction.
5   Fill your meals out with vegetables from the following list, but *don't* add fat to them unless it is within your allowance. You may only include other vegetables if they are specifically allowed in a certain meal.

Free vegetable list.   Artichokes, asparagus, aubergines, beans (green varieties only), broccoli, Brussels sprouts, cabbage, carrots, cauliflower, celery, chicory, courgettes, cucumber, lettuce, marrow, mint, mushrooms, mustard and cress, onions, parsley, peppers, radishes, spinach, spring greens, swedes, tomatoes, turnips, watercress.
6   One final, brief, but nevertheless very important point: *Do keep to the stated quantities.* Go on, make use of your kitchen scales.

Breakfasts

1 One egg, boiled and served with two crispbreads spread with butter/margarine from the allowance.
2 A half a grapefruit sweetened with artificial sweetener if desired. One egg, poached, using a little butter/margarine from the allowance and served with one slice of toasted starch-reduced bread.
3 Two rashers of back bacon, grilled and served with tomatoes cut into halves and grilled.
4 One small kipper fillet (75 g./3 oz. raw), grilled with a small amount of butter/margarine from the allowance.
5 Portion (25 g./1 oz.) of any breakfast cereal, served with one teaspoon of sugar and milk from the allowance.
6 One average sausage (50 g./2 oz. raw), well grilled and served with one rasher of streaky bacon, well grilled.

Lunches

1 Two-egg omelet, cooked in a little butter/margarine from the allowance and filled with a selection of vegetables from the free list above; one average-sized banana (150 g./6 oz. whole fruit).

2 Four fish fingers, grilled using a little butter/margarine from the allowance and served with three tablespoons of boiled peas and a teaspoon of tomato ketchup.

3 One average sausage (50 g./2 oz. raw), well grilled, served with two average kidneys, grilled by basting with a small amount of the fat from the sausage and two tomatoes cut into halves and grilled.

4 One rasher back bacon, grilled and served with liver (100 g./ 4 oz. raw), grilled by basting with a small amount of fat from the back bacon and two tablespoons of thin gravy made with very little fat.

5 A hunk of french bread (38 g. /1½ oz.) served with hard cheese (25 g./1 oz.) and one heaped teaspoon of sweet pickle.

6 Choose any of the following to make the centre piece of a salad made from vegetables in the free list above and one dessertpoon of low-calorie salad dressing:

   (a) 50 g. (2 oz.) lean pork, lamb or beef, roasted;
   (b) 75 g. (3 oz.) lean ham or chicken, cooked;
   (c) 38 g. (1½ oz.) any hard cheese, grated;
   (d) 150 g. (6 oz.) cottage cheese with chives;
   (e) two eggs, hard-boiled.

7 Make sandwiches using four slices of starch-reduced bread spread with butter/margarine from the allowance, if desired, and filled with one of the following:

   (a) one egg, hard-boiled, diced and mixed with one tomato, chopped.
   (b) 50 g. (2 oz.) of any meat paste.
   (c) 75 g. (3 oz.) cottage cheese.

8 An average-sized tin of spaghetti bolognese (approximately 181 g./7¼ oz.); one natural yoghurt (125 g./5 oz.)

9 One average slice of bread from a large loaf (38 g./1½ oz.), toasted, and topped with hard cheese (25 g./1 oz.) grated and mixed with a little milk, butter/margarine from the

allowance and a pinch of mustard powder. Serve with one heaped teaspoon of sweet chutney.

10 One average slice of bread from a large loaf (38 g./1½ oz.), toasted and topped with the contents of a small tin of baked beans (125 g./5 oz.).

11 One whole fruit yoghurt (125 g./5 oz.); one average-sized banana (150 g./6 oz. whole fruit) and apple 100 g./4 oz. whole fruit).

12 Two beefburgers, well grilled and served with three tablespoons of boiled peas and two tablespoons of thin gravy made with very little fat.

Dinners

1 *Cottage Pie*
Make a cottage pie using 75 g. (3 oz.) raw, minced beef, spices, and 75 g. (3 oz.) potato, mashed with a little butter/margarine and milk, both in addition to the allowance.

2 *Steak and Salad*
Grill 125 g. (5 oz.) of raw, lean beef steak with 6 g. (¼ oz.) butter/margarine in addition to the allowance and serve with a large mixed salad made from vegetables in the free list above.

3 *Gammon and Pineapple*
Grill 175 (7 oz.) of raw gammon with 6 g. (¼ oz.) butter/margarine in addition to the allowance and serve with two large rings of pineapple drained of excess juice.

4 *Poisson au Raisin*
Seal 150 g. (6 oz.) of any white, non-oily fish in foil, together with 75 g. (3 oz.) diced white grape halves and lemon juice. Bake until cooked (approximately thirty minutes in a moderate heat). Serve with 75 g. (3 oz.) of potato, mashed with a little butter/margarine and milk, both in addition to the allowance and two tablespoons of boiled peas. One fresh orange (100 g./4 oz. whole fruit).

5 *Cauliflower Cheese*
Take half an average-sized cauliflower (175 g./7 oz.), boil it and then cover it with a cheese sauce made from the following ingredients:

6 g. (¼ oz.) butter/margarine in addition to the allowance
6 g. (¼ oz.) flour
150 ml. (¼ pint) of milk in addition to the allowance
25 g. (1 oz.) hard cheese, grated
Seasoning and nutmeg or mace

6   *Pork Chop and Apple Sauce*
Average-sized pork chop (137 g./5½ oz. raw), well grilled and
served with one tablespoon of apple sauce and two tablespoons
of thin gravy made with very little fat.

7   *Roast Meat and Potatoes*
Roast 75 g. (3 oz.) of lean pork, lamb or beef and serve with two
small roast potato chunks (25 g./1 oz. each), some vegetables
from the free list above and two tablespoons of thin gravy made
with very little fat.

8   *Stuffed Peppers*
Top and remove the contents of two average-sized but firm
green peppers (75 g./3 oz. each). Fill each with a third of the
following mixture:
75 g. (3 oz.) chicken, roasted and sliced
25 g. (1 oz.) cottage cheese
12 g. (½ oz.) walnuts sliced
Some diced red cabbage, raw
Some bean shoots from a can
Seasoning and nutmeg
Place stuffed peppers in a tray of shallow water and bake until
cooked, in a moderate oven.

9   *Chicken in Red Wine and Orange Sauce*
Stew a small-sized joint of chicken (175 g./7 oz. raw) in water
until half cooked, then transfer to a sauce made from the
following:
6 g. (¼ oz.) flour
6 g. (¼ oz.) butter/margarine in addition to the allowance
150 ml. (¼ pint) of red wine
The juice of one small orange (75 g./3 oz. whole fruit)
Seasoning and mixed herbs.
Stew until fully cooked.

10   *Tuna or Salmon and Yoghurt Salad*
Make a large mixed salad using vegetables from the free list

above by carefully chopping all the ingredients into very small pieces and then tossing in the contents of one carton of low-fat natural yoghurt (150 ml./5 fl. oz.). Serve with either 75 g. (3 oz.) of tuna fish, drained of oil, or 125 g. (5 oz.) of steamed salmon on the bone.

11 Lamb Chops with Mint Sauce
One large lean lamb chump chop (162 g./6½ oz. raw) well grilled and served with two tablespoons of boiled peas, two tablespoons of thin gravy made with the minimum of fat and one tablespoon of mint sauce.

12 Curried Mince
Fry 75 g. (3 oz.) raw, minced beef with a level teaspoon of curry powder, a heaped teaspoon of sweet chutney, spices to taste, seasoning and the desired quantity of meat stock. Serve on a bed of 75 g. (3 oz.) boiled rice.

Daily Extras   (Each is approximately 250 Calories)

Savoury	Sweet	Liquid
175 g. (7 oz.) boiled potatoes	50 g. (2 oz.) any toffees	1½ pints mild or bitter beer
87 g. (3½ oz.) chips	62 g. (2½ oz.) boiled sweets	1 pint stout or cider
75 g. (3 oz.) lean roast pork, lamb or beef	62 g. (2½ oz.) sugar	3 pub measured (4 fl. oz. each) glasses of red or white wine
100 g. (4 oz.) lean cooked ham or chicken	38 g. (1½ oz.) milk or plain chocolate	4 pub measured (⅙ gill each) glasses of any spirit
25 g. (1 oz.) butter/margarine	3 chocolate or 4 plain biscuits	
2 average slices of bread cut from a large loaf (38 g./1½ oz. each)	1 Kit-Kat (4 fingered)	4 pub measured (⅓ gill each) glasses of any sherry
	5 whole fruit-oranges, apples or pears	3 pub measured (⅙ gill each) glasses of any liqueur
1 small packet of nuts or crisps		400 ml. (⅔ pint) of whole milk.
50 g. (2 oz.) hard cheese		

Carbohydrate – controlled

All you need do with this diet is to take good note of the carbohydrate unit values in Appendix A and make sure that you limit your intake daily to just ten carbohydrate units.

Children.   If children are following this diet and are eating their school lunch then they must allow four carbohydate units for this meal.

Fat and Protein.   If you don't seem to be having any success with this diet it could well be that you are overdoing your intake of high fatty and protein foods, so do watch out for this.

Appendix D

Balanced menus and recipes

I mentioned earlier that food which is not eaten because it is unpalatable has a nutritional value of nil. So whatever else you do, *don't* just become an expert on the theory of eating healthily. Remember that a vitally important part of good nutrition is to prepare the right foods in an appealing way; this will ensure that they are eaten and thus perform their required roles within your body.

I would say that there are five very important rules to remember whenever you are preparing a meal, whether it be a three-course dinner or food by the fireside:

1. Mix colours – for instance, white fish, cauliflower, and boiled potatoes are not the most desirable combination.
2. Mix textures – something smooth should be followed by (or eaten with) something crisp and crunchy.
3. Vary the flavours (within reason!) – for instance, lobster soup followed by lobster thermidor is not really what is wanted.
4. Cook the food for the right length of time – neither too much nor too little.
5. Spare a little time for presentation of a dish – it will be well spent.

I'm not going to give you suggestions for fireside eating because, quite frankly, these meals are normally pretty straightforward to make, but I thought it would be useful if I included some well-balanced and – none too fattening! – three-course menus. There are twelve mentioned in all; not many I know, but they should serve as a good guide for you.

Some of the meal items are very straightforward and their recipe is therefore not given; however, the more complicated ones – those that are marked with an asterisk below – are explained in full later in this section.

Menu 1   *Chestnut Soup/*Lamb en Croûte/Fresh Fruit Salad

Menu 2   Avocado with Prawns/*Chicken with Olives/ *Peaches in Orange

Menu 3   *Mushroom Soup/*Pork Chops with Nuts and Raisins/ *Orange Froth

Menu 4   *Savoury Mousse/*Hawaiian Casserole/*Golden Pears

Menu 5   *Dressed Crab/*Chicken Galantine/*Caramel Oranges

Menu 6   Melon/*Beef Stroganoff/*Meringue Cake with Damson Purée

Menu 7   *Liver pâté/*Sole Fourée/*Crème Caramel

Menu 8   *Hors D'œuvres Varié/*Blanquette of Veal/*Charlotte Russe

Menu 9   *Curried Meat/ Lychees

Menu 10   *Grapefruit with Cinnamon/ Roast Beef with all the Trimmings/*Chocolate Mousse

Menu 11   *Taramasalata/*Paupiettes de Bœuf/*Orange with Yoghurt

Menu 12   Oysters/*Duck with Cherries/Fresh Pineapple

Starters

Chestnut Soup   (for 4)

1 carrot, peeled and sliced
1 onion, peeled and sliced
25 g. (1 oz.) margarine/butter
1 (387 g./15½ oz.) can of unsweetened chestnut purée
900 ml. (1½ pints) well-flavoured stock

salt and pepper
pinch of nutmeg
1 bay leaf
the top of one bottle of milk
2 tablespoons of dry sherry, if desired

Fry carrot and onion slowly in the butter until brown. Stir in chestnut purée, stock, seasoning, nutmeg, and bay leaf. Bring to the boil, stirring all the time; then cover and simmer for about an hour.

Sieve or liquidize the soup.

Before serving, add sherry and top of the milk and gently reheat.

Serve with toast or bread.

Mushroom Soup   (for 4)

100 g. (4 oz.) mushrooms, sliced	25 g. (1 oz.) margarine or butter
600 ml. (1 pint) of stock, lightly flavoured	25 g. (1 oz.) flour
	salt and pepper
	squeeze of lemon juice
400 ml. (⅔ pint) of milk	chopped parsley to garnish

Mix together all the ingredients except the lemon juice and the parsley and bring them to the boil, whisking all the time. Then allow them to simmer for about ten minutes.

Just before serving stir in lemon juice and garnish with parsley.

Serve with french bread.

Savoury Mousse   (for 4)

150 g. (6 oz.) cream cheese	small pinch of curry powder
180 ml. (6 fl. oz.) beef consommé (concentrated)	sprigs of parsley and lemon wedges as garnishes
1 small clove garlic	

Liquidize all the ingredients (except the garnishes) together. Fill individual ramekin dishes and refrigerate until set. Garnish each dish with a sprig of parsley and lemon wedges.

Serve with hot toast.

Dressed Crab   (for 4)

4 fresh crabs	8 tablespoons mayonnaise
4 tablespoons fresh white bread crumbs	4 hard boiled eggs and chopped parsley to garnish

Prepare each of the crabs in the following way: remove the

claws and keep to one side; push the body away from the shell; remove the sixteen dead men's fingers (the breathing apparatus), the skin and the stomach. Keep dark and light meats separate.

Mix the dark meat from all the crabs with the bread crumbs and mayonnaise. Then fill the shells with alternate layers of dark and light meat.

Garnish with the slices of egg, chopped parsley and the claws.

Liver Pâté   (for 4)

200 g. (8 oz.) chicken liver
100 g. (4 oz.) margarine/ butter
1 small onion, chopped

1 garlic clove, squashed
seasonings
brandy to taste

Soften onion by frying in 25 g. (1 oz.) of the fat. Add liver and fry.

Add garlic, brandy and 50 g. (2 oz.) of melted fat. Liquidize. Spread smoothly in four individual dishes.

Cool, and pour a layer of fat still remaining on top of each dish (this will keep the pâté soft). Serve with toast.

Hors D'oeuvres Varié

Six varieties of foods are usually served, and it is important to get a good mixture of colours and textures.

Some suggestions for the different varieties are shown opposite.

Grapefruit with Cinnamon   (for 4)

2 whole grapefruit, cut into halves

4 heaped teaspoons brown sugar
cinnamon

Gently free the flesh from the skin of each of the grapefruit halves.

Sprinkle one heaped teaspoon of brown sugar and cinnamon on top of each and then place under a hot grill for 5–10 minutes.

Food	Garnish
Cauliflower heads with orange slices	Chopped chives or parsley sprigs
Tomato and onion rings	Chopped chives or parsley sprigs
Sweetcorn	Green and red peppers
Asparagus	Lemon
Vegetable salad Potato salad	Chopped parsley or stuffed/black olives, or pickled walnuts
Egg mayonnaise	Anchovies
Grated carrot Beetroot in soured cream	Chopped chives
Salami slices Smoked sausage slices Ham rolled round pineapple	Radishes or nuts
Sardines Pilchards Tuna, flaked Prawns Sprats	Lemon slices
Salmon rolled around asparagus tips	
Rice cooked and mixed with dressing or mayonnaise and crisp vegetables	
Slices of meat or nuts	

Taramasalata   (for 4)

1 thin slice of white bread from a large loaf, into fine crumbs
200 g. (8 oz.) smoked cod's roe
1 small potato, boiled and mashed

1 clove of garlic
juice of half a lemon
1 tablespoon olive oil
parsley sprigs or olives to garnish

Blend together the bread crumbs, cod's roe, mashed potato and garlic. Then mix in the oil.

Place the mixture in four individual dishes garnished with the parsley or olives and serve with toast.

Main courses

Lamb en Croûte   (for 4)

1 best end neck of lamb

egg, beaten for glazing

Stuffing

1 small onion, finely chopped	3 tablespoons of chopped
6 g. (¼ oz.) margarine/butter	apricots
3 tablespoons of fresh white	1 egg to bind
bread crumbs	

Flaky pastry

200 g. (8 oz.) plain flour	150 g. (6 oz.) margarine/
½ level teaspoon of salt	butter and lard mixed
7 tablespoons of cold water	

To make flaky pastry   Divide the fat into four equal portions. Sieve the flour and salt together and rub in a quarter of the fat (keep the remaining fat cool). Add water and work the ingredients into a dough. Knead on a floured surface for about 2 minutes.

Sprinkle with flour and then leave to rest in a polythene bag for about 15–20 minutes in a refrigerator. Then roll out pastry into an oblong and dot the top two-thirds of one side with a quarter of the fat.

Fold the bottom third up and the top third down to cover the fat. Seal the edges with a rolling pin.

Place in a polythene bag in the refrigerator as before and then repeat the above process with the two other quarters of the fat.

Finally, put the pastry in a refrigerator for 15 minutes before using.

To make Lamb en Croûte   Remove bones from the lamb.

Make the stuffing by lightly frying the onions in the fat and then mix them with the rest of the ingredients. Spread the mixture across the inside of the deboned meat.

Roll the lamb into a cylindrical shape. Roll out the pastry and place the prepared lamb within it. Then fold the pastry over the meat in order to completely cover it.

Decorate with pastry leaves made from the trimmings. Glaze with some beaten egg.

Bake for 15 minutes in a hot oven (200°C/425°F or gas mark 7) and then finish cooking in a moderate oven (180°C/350°F or gas mark 4) for a further 20 minutes or until fully cooked.

Serve with green vegetables and boiled potatoes.

Chicken with Olives   (for 4)

1 1.3 kg. (3 lb.) chicken cut into pieces
4 tablespoons olive oil
2 large onions, sliced
1 clove of garlic, crushed
400 g. (16 oz.) canned tomatoes
12 green olives, sliced

100 g. (4 oz.) carrots, diced
1 thick slice of white bread minus crusts, into bread crumbs
150 ml. ($\frac{1}{4}$ pint) dry white wine
salt and pepper

Fry the chicken pieces in three-fourths of the olive oil until golden brown, then remove from the pan and keep hot.

Fry the onions and garlic. Add the drained tomatoes and stock. When the mixture starts to simmer put in chicken joints and season.

Cover the pan and simmer for about half an hour until the chicken is tender. Remove the chicken and keep hot in a serving dish.

Add diced carrots and bread crumbs to ingredients in the frying pan and cook for a couple of minutes longer. Then liquidize this mixture, return it to the pan add wine and sliced olives and reheat.

Pour this sauce over chicken. Serve with rice and a green vegetable or salad.

Pork Chops with Nuts and Raisins

4 pork chops
50 g. (2 oz.) whole almonds
50 g. (2 oz.) raisins
25 g. (1 oz.) margarine/ butter
1 green pepper, diced

300 ml. ($\frac{1}{2}$ pint) of stock, lightly flavoured
the grated rind of 1 lemon
1 bay leaf
salt and pepper
2 tablespoons tomato purée

Grill the pork chops for about 10 minutes on each side and then place in a serving dish.

Soften the pepper in the fat (about 5 minutes). Add the rest of the ingredients to the pepper and simmer for about 10 minutes.

Remove the bay leaf and pour this mixture over the chops in the serving dish.

Serve with tomatoes, green vegetables and boiled potatoes.

Hawaiian Casserole   (for 4)

300 g. (12 oz.) ham, cooked and diced
50 g. (2 oz.) raisins
75 g. (3 oz.) pineapple cubes

1 medium-sized onion sliced in rings
1 medium green pepper sliced in rings

To make syrup
120 ml. (4 fl. oz.) pineapple syrup
50 g. (2 oz.) brown sugar
60 ml. (2 fl. oz.) vinegar
2 tablespoons cornstarch

2 teaspoons dry mustard
¼ teaspoon salt
1 tablespoon each of Worcester and soy sauce

Prepare the syrup by bringing all the relevant ingredients to the boil and then allowing them to simmer, very gently, until the syrup forms.

Place the onions, pineapple cubes, green pepper, raisins and ham in a serving dish in layers and cover the whole with the syrup.

Cover and cook in a moderate oven (180°C/350°F or gas mark 4) for about 40 minutes.

Serve with peas and sweetcorn and baked potatoes.

Chicken Galantine   (for 4)

1 1.3 kg. (3 lb.) chicken

Stuffing
200 g. (8 oz.) sausage meat
2 rashers of streaky bacon
25 g. (1 oz.) mixed nuts, chopped
2 teaspoons parsley, chopped

100 g. (4 oz.) mushrooms, diced
1 small onion, sliced
25 g. (1 oz.) fresh white bread crumbs
salt and pepper

Bone chicken (start from the base *not* the breast, and be careful not to pierce the skin). Flatten the meat and spread with the stuffing.

Roll up in a neat shape, wrap in greased greaseproof paper and foil and cook in a moderately hot oven (200°C/400°F or gas mark 6) allowing 25 minutes to the pound.

Serve hot or cold (if so, it is nice glazed in aspic jelly) with a mixed salad and boiled potatoes.

Beef Stroganoff   (for 4)

400 g. (16 oz.) fillet or rump
   steak
1 onion, chopped
300 ml. (½ pint) ordinary or
   soured cream
200 g. (8 oz.) mushrooms,
   sliced
100 g. (4 oz.) margarine/
   butter

juice of 2 lemons
2 tablespoons of sherry or
   brandy
2 level dessertspoons chopped
   parsley
1 heaped tablespoon of
   seasoned flour
salt and pepper

Lightly fry the mushrooms and onions in half of the fat and then remove them from the pan. Now, using the other half of the fat very quickly fry the steak which has been cut into small chunks – against the grain of the meat – and dipped in the seasoned flour. This will seal the pieces of meat. Now, place all the ingredients together and stir until very hot – be careful not to boil.

Serve with rice and mixed vegetables.

Sole Fourée   (for 4)

4 soles (this recipe works
   equally well as for plaice)
50 g. (2 oz.) margarine/butter

150 g. (6 oz.) fresh bread
   crumbs

Filling

25 g. (1 oz.) margarine/
   butter
25 g. (1 oz.) flour
300 ml. (½ pint) milk

100 g. (4 oz.) prawns
100 g. (4 oz.) mushrooms,
   chopped and lightly fried
2 tablespoons cream

Remove dark skin, lift the fillets on both sides and remove backbone.

Make up filling by preparing a sauce from the butter, flour, milk and cream; and then by adding the prawns and the mushrooms. Fill the cavity of each fish with the prawn mixture.

Brush well with melted butter and cover with bread crumbs. Cook in a moderate oven (180°C/350°F or gas mark 4) for about 30 minutes.

Serve with creamed potatoes and green vegetables.

Blanquette of Veal   (for 4)

800 g. (32 oz.) pie veal or 400 g. (16 oz.) best trimmings	½ level teaspoon salt
	pepper
	2 cloves
1½ litres (2½ pints) water – approximately	1 bay leaf
	thyme
12 small onions	mace
2 carrots, finely chopped	

Sauce

25 g. (1 oz.) butter	2 egg yolks
25 g. (1 oz.) flour	2 tablespoons cream
Add some of the liquid from the meat	the juice of 1 lemon
	sprig parsley, finely chopped
100 g. (4 oz.) mushrooms, sliced	

Cut meat into 2½ cm. (1 in.) cubes. Place in pan with salt, lemon and water and bring to the boil slowly. Then drain and rinse.

Return meat to the rinsed pan with the prepared carrot, onion, herbs and 600 ml. (1 pint) water. Cover and simmer for an hour till tender. Strain off and keep liquid (about 300–400 ml. or ½–¾ pints). Discard the vegetables and herbs.

Make the sauce by melting the butter in a saucepan, adding the flour and cooking for 1–2 minutes. Then add the water which has been kept from cooking the meat and boil the mixture for 3 minutes. Then blend the egg yolks with the cream and add gradually to the sauce. Add lemon juice, season and replace meat. Heat gently for 5 minutes, *do not boil.*

Serve with carrots and boiled potatoes.

Curried Meat   (for 4)

400 g. (16 oz.) meat (beef, lamb, or chicken), sliced
25 g. (1 oz.) flour
1 onion, chopped
1 tablespoon of curry powder (level = mild curry, rounded = medium curry)
25 g. (1 oz.) margarine/ butter
lemon juice to taste
1 tablespoon black treacle
1 tablespoon red currant jelly or apricot jam

1 tablespoon chutney
600 ml. (1 pint) stock, well flavoured
1 bay leaf
1 teaspoon parsley, chopped
1 clove garlic, crushed
25 g. (1 oz.) sultanas
some black peppercorns
sliced apple
chillies
tumeric   } optional
ginger
coconut

Melt butter and add curry powder, onions, flour, meat and then the stock – bit by bit.

Add all the other ingredients, bring to the boil and then simmer the mixture until the meat is cooked.

Serve with rice and a vegetable curry (made in a similar way to the above, but using vegetables instead of the meat).

Paupiettes de Boeuf   (for 4)

4 thin slices of buttock steak, beaten between greaseproof paper

Forcemeat
¼ onion or shallot
3 green olives
50 g. (2 oz.) sausage meat

half a beaten egg
pinch of thyme/pepper/salt
a few bread crumbs

Mirepoix

2 onions, chopped	25 g. (1 oz.) bacon
2 carrots, chopped	2 tablespoons tomato purée
celery, chopped	enough brown stock to just
25 g. (1 oz.) margarine/	cover the vegetables
butter	

Remove fat from the bacon, chop the lean and lightly fry. Beat steak and divide into quarters. Trim into oblong shapes, add the trimmings to the forcemeat.

Mix together the ingredients for the forcemeat and then spread the resultant mixture on to the oblong of meat. Roll up the meat with the sides slightly tucked in – shape them to ensure that they are all the same size – and then tie them in two or three places.

To make the mirepoix.   Melt the butter, add chopped bacon, and vegetables, and then sauté until the fat is absorbed. Place in the base of an oven-proof dish and lay the prepared paupiettes on top.

Cook for 1 hour in a very moderately hot oven (170°C/375°F or gas mark 3).

Serve with piped creamed potatoes and carrots/green vegetables.

Duck with Cherries   (for 4)

1 2 kg. (4½ lb) ready-to-cook duck

The sauce

3 tablespoons sugar	about 40 black cherries,
25 g. (1 oz.) arrowroot,	soaked in a mixture of 1
blended with 2 table-	tablespoon of lemon juice,
spoons of port	3 tablespoons of brandy,
150 ml. (¼ pint) red wine	and 2 tablespoons sugar
vinegar	for about half an hour
450 ml. (¾ pint) strong brown	
stock, made from the duck	
giblets	

Roast the duck in a moderate oven (180°C/350°F or gas mark 4) for about 1 hour 20 minutes.

Prepare the sauce by boiling the sugar and the vinegar together until they form a syrup. Immediately remove from the heat and pour in a quarter of the stock. Simmer for a minute and then add the rest of the stock.

Beat in the arrowroot mixture and simmer for 3–4 minutes. Add the juices from the roasted meat to the sauce, and then add this whole mixture to the cherries.

Very gently heat the resultant combination for 3–4 minutes. Remove the cherries from the sauce and place around the duck. Boil the remaining ingredients until thickened slightly. Spoon a bit of this sauce on to the meat and serve the rest separately.

Serve with roast potatoes and peas.

Desserts

Peaches in Orange   (for 4)

8 peach halves minus the syrup	25 g. (1 oz.) castor sugar
12 g. (½ oz.) margarine/ butter	6 tablespoons of any orange liqueur

Gently fry peach halves in the fat and then sprinkle with the sugar and allow to caramelize.

Finally, add the liqueur and set alight.

Orange Froth   (for 4)

juice of 2 oranges	12 g. (½ oz.) gelatine
juice of half a lemon	3 large eggs
4 tablespoons cold water	75 g. (3 oz.) castor sugar

Dissolve the gelatine.

Separate the eggs, add two-thirds of the sugar to the yolks and whisk until pale. Then add the fruit juice and, finally, the dissolved gelatine, stirring all the time. Leave to set, giving it an occasional whisk.

When set, whisk together the egg whites and the remaining sugar and then fold into the orange mixture.

Place in a serving bowl and leave to set firmly.

Golden Pears (for 4)

4 firm pears, peeled but kept
  whole and with stalks
  still in place
2 small oranges, 1 for the
  garnish

1 level teaspoon of cinnamon
  (powdered)
50 g. (2 oz.) brown sugar
150 ml. ($\frac{1}{4}$ pint) apple juice
1 level tablespoon arrowroot
8 cloves

Place the pears in a large ovenproof dish and add the grated
rind and juice from 1 orange. Then add the sugar, cloves and
apple juice.

Cover with foil but keep the pears sticking through so that
they remain upright.

Place in a moderate oven (180°C/350°F or gas mark 4) for
1–1$\frac{1}{2}$ hours until the pears are tender. Transfer to a serving dish.
Strain the liquid and thicken with arrowroot.

Decorate with orange pieces and then pour over the thickened
mixture.

Serve hot or cold.

Caramel Oranges (for 4)

4 oranges, peeled and thinly
  sliced into circles
150 g. (6 oz.) granulated
  sugar

$\frac{3}{4}$ teacup cold water
1 teacup hot water

Dissolve sugar in the cold water by applying a gentle heat and
then bring to the boil rapidly until the mixture begins to caramelize. Do not allow it to get dark brown. Then, very carefully
holding the pan with a cloth, add the hot water and stir into
the caramel. Pour over the orange slices in a dish and allow
to cool.

Meringue Cake with Damson Purée (for 4)

4 egg whites
200 g. (8 oz.) castor sugar

300 ml. ($\frac{1}{2}$ pint) of double
  cream
damson purée, as desired

Whip the egg whites to a firm snow. Add 1 tablespoon of sugar and whisk a further minute. Fold in the rest of the sugar using a metal spoon.

Lightly oil three rounds of greaseproof paper (approx. 20 cm./ 8 in. in diameter). Spread the meringue mixture evenly on each round, slide on to a baking sheet and dry in a cool oven (140°C/ 275°F or gas mark 1) until firm.

Cool and peel off the paper. Sandwich the meringue together with whipped cream and serve with damson purée.

Crème Caramel   (for 4)

75 g. (3 oz.) castor sugar	2 egg yolks
3 tablespoons water	2 tablespoons sugar
squeeze of lemon juice	600 ml. (1 pint) milk
2 whole eggs	

Dissolve the castor sugar, water and lemon juice together under a gentle heat, and then bring to the boil rapidly until the mixture begins to caramelize. Do not allow it to get dark brown.

Remove from the heat and pour into a warmed greased soufflé dish, making sure that the mixture coats the whole basin.

Beat the eggs and remaining sugar with a fork; heat the milk until just about boiling and then pour on to the beaten eggs. Mix this mixture with the caramel, having first strained it.

Cook by standing in a baking tin filled with enough water to half coat the sides of the soufflé dish. Cover with some foil and bake in a slow oven (150°C/300°F or gas mark 2) for about an hour until completely set.

Allow the sweet to cool before turning out on to a serving dish.

Serve with heated banana slices.

Charlotte Russe   (for 4)

1 packet sponge or boudoir fingers	1 lemon jelly

Filling

150 ml. (¼ pint) any fruit   lemon juice
   puree   12 g. (½ oz.) gelatine
150 ml. (¼ pint) cream   3½ tablespoons of water
150 ml. (¼ pint) egg custard,
   i.e. 2 tablespoons milk,
   2 eggs, sugar to taste

Garnish

cream   chopped nuts
sliced jelly

Surround the sides of an average-sized soufflé dish with the sponge biscuits in an upright position, next to each other. Cut off the top part of the biscuits so that they don't protrude above the edge of the dish.

Make up half a packet of jelly and pour it into the bottom of the prepared dish. Leave to set.

Beat the eggs, milk and sugar together. Then stir over hot water until thickened — it will also thicken as it cools. To the cold custard add the fruit purée, cream, gelatine (which has already been dissolved in the water) and lemon juice.

Pour the above filling over the set jelly.

Garnish with a small amount of cream, some of the remaining jelly cubes (sliced) and finally some chopped nuts.

Chocolate Mousse   (for 4)

100 g. (4 oz.) plain chocolate   2 tablespoons brandy
4 eggs, separated   2 tablespoons sugar

Garnish
4 whole almonds

Put chocolate into a basin and place over a pan of hot water. Stir until the chocolate is soft. Add the egg yolks and the sugar and beat until thick. Add the brandy and beat again. Take the basin out of the pan and fold in the stiffly beaten egg whites.

Spoon into four individual glasses, and top each with an almond when set.

Orange with Yoghurt   (for 4)

juice of 2 oranges	4 cartons of natural yoghurt
25 g. (1 oz.) sugar	the flesh of 4 oranges, cut into pieces

Dissolve the sugar in the orange juice by heating gently, then bring rapidly to the boil and keep boiling just until the mixture turns syrupy. Pour into 4 individual serving dishes. Allow to cool completely.

Add the yoghurt, which will have been well beaten, to the mixture in each of the serving dishes.

Decorate each with some of the orange pieces.

You may be wondering why I have included so many sweet ideas. I have more than once been accusingly asked, just as I was about to tuck into something quite delightful, 'You're not going to eat that, are you?' as though it was the worst possible sin that I, as a nutritionist, could commit.

The big point to remember here is that so long as I keep my first helping to a reasonable size and don't have a second or a third, then there is absolutely no reason why I (or you, for that matter) should not have a little bit of what we fancy.

Appendix E

Suggested books for further reading

General nutrition

The Value of Food, P. Fisher and A. E. Bender, Oxford University Press, 1975.

Manual of Nutrition, the Ministry of Agriculture Fisheries and Food, Her Majesty's Stationery Office, 1976.

The Second Book of Food and Nutrition, Wendy Matthews and Dilys Wells, Home Economics and The Flour Advisory Bureau, 1976.

This Nutrition Business, John Yudkin, Davis-Poynter, 1976.

Special topics

Why Additives?, British Nutrition Foundation, Forbes Publications, 1977.

The Which Guide to Slimming, Consumers' Association, 1977.

The Joy of Slimming, Margaret Allen, Hodder and Stoughton, 1976.

This Slimming Business, John Yudkin, Penguin Books Ltd., 1974.

Cooking for your Heart's Content, Katie Dyson, Hutchinson and Co. Ltd., 1976.

Index